THE BODY IN NURSING

TWENTY ONE DAY LOAN

This item is to be returned on
or before the date stamped below

1 8 FEB 1999
CANCELLED

1 5 MAR 1999
CANCELLED

1 0 NOV 2000

1 1 JAN 2001

1 2 JAN 2006

UNIVERSITY OF PLYMOUTH

EXETER LIBRARY

Tel: (01392) 475049
This book is subject to recall if required by another reader
Books may be renewed by phone
CHARGES WILL BE MADE FOR OVERDUE BOOKS

WITHDRAWN
FROM
UNIVERSITY OF ... H

D1440507

THE BODY IN NURSING

Jocalyn Lawler

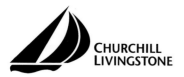

CHURCHILL
LIVINGSTONE

CHURCHILL LIVINGSTONE
An imprint of Pearson Professional (Australia) Pty Ltd

Kings Gardens
95 Coventry Street
South Melbourne VIC 3205
Australia

Pearson Professional offices in Hong Kong, Singapore, Japan, USA, Canada, India, United
Kingdom and Europe.

Text and design copyright © Pearson Professional (Australia) Pty Ltd 1997
Photographs (reproduced on cover and in text by permission) copyright © Peter Short 1997

Conditions of Sale
All rights reserved. Except under the conditions described in the Copyright Act 1968 of
Australia and subsequent amendments, no part of this publication may be reproduced, stored
in a retrieval system or transmitted in any form or by any means, electronic, mechanical,
photocopying, recording or otherwise, without the prior permission of the copyright owner.

No responsibility for loss occasioned to any person acting or refraining from action as a result
of the material in this publication can be accepted by the Author or Publishers.

First published 1997

Edited by Mignon Turpin
Cover designed by Sylvia Witte
Photography by Peter Short
Printed in Singapore

National Library of Australia
Cataloguing-in-Publication data

The body in nursing.

ISBN 0 443 05250 6.

1. Nurse and patient. 2. Nursing - Psychological aspects.
3. Mind and body. I. Lawler, Jocalyn.

610.73

UNIVERSITY OF PLYMOUTH
LIBRARY SERVICES

Item
No.   9003692095

Class
No.   616. 0019   LAW

Contl
No.   0443 052506

The
publisher's
policy is to use
paper manufactured
from sustainable forests

Contents

Contributors

JOCALYN LAWLER RN, PhD
Professor of Nursing, Faculty of Nursing, The University of Sydney

PETER SHORT RN, BA, MPH
Lecturer, University of Technology, Sydney and doctoral candidate at the Univeristy of Sydney

JUDITH PARKER RN, PhD
Professor of Nursing, School of Nursing, La Trobe University

IRENA MADJAR RN, PhD
Professor of Nursing, Faculty of Nursing, The University of Newcastle

TRUDY RUDGE RN, BA (HONS)
Lecturer, University of South Australia and doctoral candidate at La Trobe University

PAMELA VAN DER RIET RN, BA, MED
Lecturer, La Trobe University and doctoral candidate at James Cook University

JUDY LUMBY RN, PhD
E.M. Lane Professor of Nursing, The University of Sydney and Concord Hospital

STUART NEWMAN RN, BED(N), MHP
Health Services Manager, Nimbin Hospital, and doctoral candidate at The University of Sydney

MAUREEN BOUGHTON RN, BED(N)
Lecturer, Faculty of Nursing, and doctoral candidate at The University of Sydney

JAN HORSFALL RN, PhD
Associate Professor of Nursing, Faculty of Nursing, The University of Sydney

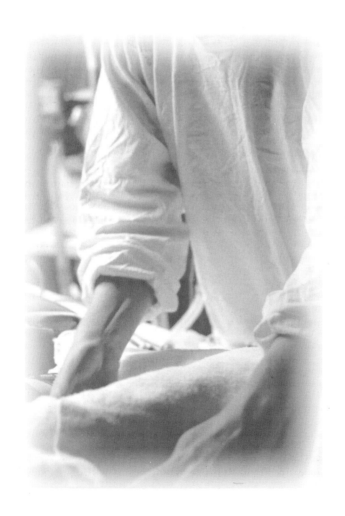

Locating the body in nursing: an introduction

Jocalyn Lawler

There is no single moment at which this book began. There were, however, a couple of events that have been significant. One such event occurred in July 1993 at the International Council of Nursing meeting in Madrid, Spain. Perhaps we were affected by the simmering mid-summer heat, or maybe we were more inclined to find our common points of interest because so much around us was relatively unfamiliar. Judy Parker, Irena Madjar and I decided in Madrid to present a symposium on our various works on the body and embodiment at the Sigma Theta Tau International conference to be held the following year in Sydney, Australia.

In our approach to the symposium we wanted to stimulate debate and discussion in this area, rather than present 'finished' works or highly ordered argument. That would have been premature in any event, because much of our work on embodiment, the body, and nursing is characterised by a sense of feeling our way, of skirting the boundaries and the mysteries of new terrain and new ways of working with the stuff that is nursing's epistemic and methodological spaces. Our major intention was to attempt to locate the body and embodiment more centrally among the concerns of nursing research, thinking and scholarship because, to us, the body and embodiment were already centrally located among the daily concerns of practising nurses.

While we each were aware of the others' works prior to the Madrid meeting, we had not previously attempted to bring our ideas together simultaneously in time and place. Also, we were encouraged by the knowledge that among us we had a number of doctoral students whose works focused variously on issues of embodiment and its location in the epistemic project of nursing. It seemed — to borrow a term from the scientists — that we had reached a 'critical mass' of scholars in the field such that we could attract an audience for a symposium. Our judgement proved correct and the response to the symposium exceeded our expectations; it was lively, well attended (indeed the venue had to be moved to accommodate the larger audience) and stimulated considerable discussion.

Our three papers from that symposium, in revised and extended forms, appear in this volume as Chapters 2, 3 and 4 — their original order. While they have been revised and extended as a result of the discussions that flowed from the symposium and further work, they are not finished works in the normal sense.

We are joined in this collection by seven of our Australian colleagues. Their essays variously address the theme of how and why the body and embodiment — as substantive concerns of nursing's episteme — can be approached, theorised, discussed and articulated. More importantly, they offer a range of ways in which we can locate the body and embodiment among the scholarly concerns of nursing. Many different starting points are apparent in this collection, yet each of the essays converges or coincides with the others, highlighting commonalties, issues, debates, questions and uncertainties. The project on the body and embodiment has been a very recent development in the academy and this is true also for nursing. The essays in this collection, therefore, are very much works in progress, and they are necessarily unfinished and often asking more questions than they answer.

This was not an orchestrated and choreographed collection of essays, nor has it been 'homogenised' in the editorial process. The authors have been free to develop their work independently of their fellow contributors; the result is a 'collection' in every sense of the word. As the editor, I was anxious not to get in the way of the more free-ranging ways in which scholars are addressing the body in nursing, offering guidance only in circumstances where authors tended to discuss in detail theoretical points that could be repeated in other chapters.

Peter Short's pictures, which appear on the cover and throughout the book, add a dimension to ways in which nurses might study and represent the body and embodiment. They are unusual and poignant reminders that there is much in nursing practice that defies, transcends, and avoids language. These pictures also highlight the horrors and abjections that often surround the human body as it becomes a site for medical and nursing encounters and a location for embodied struggles.

Judy Parker's chapter draws on her work on the body and embodiment that extends over almost two decades. There is, consequently, both great depth and scope in her chapter, as well as signs that she is entering into new and exciting territory. Judy's work in this field (and others) has had far reaching influence both in Australia and internationally. In this chapter she moves into the terrain of the temporospatial and (post)modern body, taking us into exciting new territory and opening new lines of inquiry and thought for nursing.

Chapter 4 is an extension of work that I began in the early 1980s and which is on-going. My major project concerns the multiple ways in which nursing is silenced and rendered invisible. I have been concerned to unpack the pattern of social responses and practices surrounding the body and reasons why it has been simultaneously obvious and yet obscure. In this chapter, my focus has shifted to more overtly address the nature of the discourses that draw us toward the objectification of people, health and illness in our search to understand them and to work in health care. My chapter is also an(other) attempt to address the limitations and dangers of economically driven discourses for human(e) disciplines.

Irena Madjar's chapter has its origins in her doctoral work with patients' experiences of pain, particularly that which is clinically inflicted — imposed as a necessary condition for recovery and renewal as an embodied 'other'. Her work is phenomenologically oriented and located firmly in the clinical domain of the nurse. Irena's work invites us to look beyond the more conventional wisdom about pain and suffering and enter the world of the suffering 'other' and the space that nurses and their patients jointly experience and inhabit.

Trudy Rudge's essay also draws on data from the clinical field of nursing. She focuses her attention more firmly on the boundedness and boundaries of the body and embodiment, particularly as they are experienced by patients with burns. Her work, and that of Irena Madjar, complement each other in substance and style. In many ways Trudy's work is characteristic of much contemporary doctoral work among Australian nurses — it is well grounded in classic texts, yet it moves us into an intellectual space that is rich in metaphors, meanings and experiences. There is much in this chapter that will reflect practitioners' everyday work.

Pamela van der Riet takes up the issue of medicalised power as it is mediated by technologies. She positions technologies both in the mechanical and discursive domains. This is very much an unfinished work because there are so few attempts in the nursing literature that address the troublesome issues of how one provides highly technologised care while also realising that humans are the focus of such attention.

Judy Lumby overtly addresses the issues that affect gender, being and illness. In particular she examines the ways in which these concepts are indivisible during episodes of illness. In this particular chapter, Judy takes up a major theme that has characterized her research — feminism and the feminized nature of much of the work and issues that nurses and women deal with every day. Judy's chapter draws from her doctoral project as well as work that is in progress.

Stuart Newman takes a courageous look at masculinity (masculinities) and the male body, with particular emphasis on developing lines of inquiry in nursing. He reviews the current status of thinking about the relationships among maleness, masculinities, men's bodies, embodiment and men's health. Like most of the chapters in this collection, his work draws on his doctoral project that is exploring the apparently (un)gendered nature of many nursing practices and their relationship to men's experiences of nursing care and illness.

Maureen Boughton also draws on her doctoral work on women's experience of premature menopause to speculate on the relationships among biology, self and experience. She highlights some of the issues that are confronted by individuals as they struggle to reconcile their biological bodies with their embodied selves among an array of social influences that imbue the body with particular meanings.

The last chapter in this collection is Jan Horsfall's provocative analysis of the mind/body divide that is characteristic of much thinking in psychiatry and much of the practice of psychiatric nursing. In many ways, the issues that are raised in this chapter appear to be both obvious yet strangely ignored among scholars in this area.

There is no singular paradigmatic position that characterises the works in this collection, though many of them are influenced by various aspects of what we have come to call the postmodern period. One of the most interesting aspects of this collection is that although many of the authors began from very different starting points, they have converged on several key issues on which they appear to agree: that the body and embodiment are obvious and necessary locations for scholarly works in the discipline of nursing; that these are the locations of some of the most severely felt tensions between biomedical-scientific constructs of health care practice and lived experience; and that the epistemological fields that enlighten us about the physical body are often at odds with fields of inquiry that inform us about the lived body and the experienced world of the 'other'.

This book is published at a time when there is an explosion of works dealing with varying aspects of the body and embodiment. This trend is particularly apparent within disciplines that are explicitly concerned with human social life, such as sociology and feminism (see for example, Bordo 1993, Connell 1995, Grosz 1994, Grosz and Probyn 1996) and there is also much transdisciplinary and interdisciplinary work in this field (for example, Lalvani 1996, Raschke 1996).

In many ways, the focus on the human body — as it is represented, studied, conceptualised, imaged, imagined, re-made, and experienced — typifies the postmodern period in which the apparent divisions between subject and object are themselves the primary focus for discussion and debate. Just as the postmodern period has been typified, among other things, by a dismantling of boundaries, so too it has been typified by explorations of the ways in which things are interconnected; this is particularly so in the domain of the human body and human experiences in health, illness and health care.

Nursing has had a long and continuing struggle with the apparent but artefactual separability of subject and object — between what can be felt and experienced as distinct from what can be seen, measured and expressed in words. In recent decades this debate has taken shape in the form of debate as to whether nursing is an art or a science, a unique body of knowledge in its own right or an applied discipline that draws predominantly from other (more 'pure') disciplines. These debates, which remain unresolved, have an irreconcilable quality about them perhaps because they have their origins in the false premise that it is possible to make a clear and sustainable distinction between the ways we understand the scientific-objective world and the experienced-subjective world.

This collection, while it in part is a critique of ways of thinking about and researching nursing, also is an attempt to focus on the epistemic underpinnings of nursing in so far as that concerns the embodied experience of humans. The works also draw significantly from philosophical writings; that is not to say that this is a book about philosophies of nursing (as attractive as that notion is), rather, it is about ways in which we can enrich our thinking about nursing and our practice and research by considering fundamental questions about what it is to be human, and what it is to be ill or distressed or to need the skills and understanding of nurses.

This is a different kind of text from those which many have come to expect in nursing. And it differs from the kinds of genres that we have seen written for a nursing audience. Much of nursing's scholarly writings are constructed within the frames of reference of 'others'. Or they necessarily are 'how to' books designed for safe practice. Much has been documented in nursing in response to external threats. Much of that work has focused on ways in which others might understand what we do. Other works have focused on how we might understand and identify ourselves and our selves — as a precursor to understanding our relationship(s) to the 'other', particularly in our practice and research. This book is about how we might understand an important and central part of the knowledge that informs nursing practice, thought, research and the space(s) we occupy in health care.

REFERENCES

Bordo S 1993 Unbearable weight: feminism, western culture and the body. University of California Press, Berkeley

Connell R W 1995 Masculinities. Allen & Unwin, Sydney

Grosz E 1994 Volatile bodies: towards a corporeal feminism. Allen & Unwin, Sydney

Grosz E & Probyn E 1996 Sexy bodies: the strange carnalities of feminism. Routledge, London

Lalvani S 1996 Photography, vision, and the production of modern bodies. State University of New York, Albany

Raschke C A 1996 Fire and roses: postmodernity and thought of the body. State University of New York, Albany

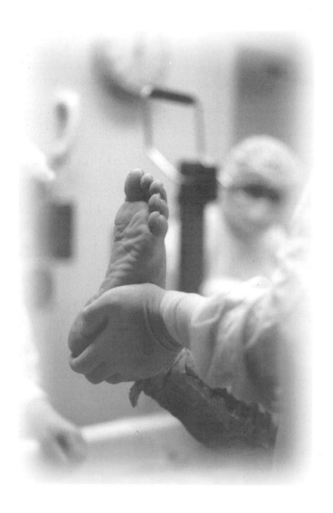

2

Picturing the body in nursing

Peter Short

Photography is an ubiquitous aspect of everyday life. Modern life is, at times, like a stroll through a continuous exhibition of photographic imagery. Advertising pictures, personal snapshots, book covers, magazines and newspapers assail us with photographic messages (Tagg 1988:34). We experience the world through images of it.

Photography is a cultural practice that provides meaning. In the developed world, it is conventional, structured and despite the 'bourgeois folklore' (Sekula 1982:86) that it is inherently truthful, it aids in manufacturing appearances. Photography has been used to threaten *and* support the status quo, and photographs have been given the status of legal documents.

Many people consider photographs only as a means of decorating an otherwise totally verbal publication, they do not realise the amount of information a photograph can provide, most of which is unavailable from other sources (Rudisill 1982). While a photograph may show, for instance, a surgical operation being performed, it also gives information about notions of sterility, relationships between the participants, the technology used and much more; this is not to say, however, that photography can be taken at face value.

Photographs tell stories and, like other texts, their meanings are contestable; the range of possible readings, and therefore meanings, depends upon the work done by the reader (Hall 1980:128–138). Context can also determine meaning. For example, a documentary photograph showing nurses at work in 1995 can, when shown in the year 2050, assume the title 'art'. In Susan Sontag's (1979:21) view, time positions all photographs at the level of art. The same pictures could be used to determine work practices that could improve 'efficiency' among nursing (in terms of a time-and-motion study) or as evidence for a demographic study of nurses. The pictures in this book have a meaning different from what was originally intended.

Photographs have been made in hospital since the 'invention' of photography in 1839 because of its alliances with medicine. Clinical medical images depicted the body through its lesions, deformities, human types and medical treatments. Commemorative medical images showed the body as secondary to new treatments or to the meetings of eminent medical men (and they were mostly men). Photographic technology is extensively used in diagnostics and images continue to be made of 'interesting' cases of pathology for teaching, research and commemoration.

In spite of the alliance between medicine and photography, we are rarely shown what happens to people in hospitals. Medical images tend to remain just that; they usually reside in archives in hospitals or universities for the use of staff only. Television serials provide images of the ideal, as opposed to the real. In these, people with severe, life-threatening wounds retain a certain look of Hollywood glamour. The sick body, by and large, remains unseen. In society where the ideal body is young, slim and undamaged and where bodies are exposed for casual view in magazines, newspapers and on the beach, the sight of the injured, disfigured or dysfunctional body identifies it as a 'pathological other' (Gilman 1988:4) and precludes its visibility.

Within hospitals, though, a line is clearly drawn between those who can look with impunity and those who cannot. The patient/client's body is available for examination, inspection and discussion by staff but not by casual visitors from 'the outside'. Staff confidentiality is offered within the frame of the caring relationship while non-clinical photography has an explicit aim of (relatively) public exposure. Staff confidentiality offers the patient/client some, albeit limited, control over their bodies. Non-clinical photographs taken while in hospital threaten the person's loss of control over what is seen, when, how and by whom.

Foucault (1980:155) argued that people internalise external sources of discipline, making themselves, instead, self-disciplined. Self-discipline over bodily exposure of sickness, dysfunction and injury, combined with the inherent threat of exposure offered by photography, makes photography in hospital, at times, frustrating. Having a sick body is not a value neutral experience because, as Gilman (1988:7) says, symbolic fictions create meanings for every type of disease or dysfunction. Increasing use of science and technology has not lessened the blame heaped on sick people for their illness(es). Society does not, as Sontag (1979) believed it should, see disease simply as disease, but as metaphors; these metaphors are themselves value-laden, symbolic and constructed, in part, by imagery.

In addition to symbolic fictions that are captured on film, there are fictions about nurses and their work. Because of a lack of imagery about nurses working with injured, disfigured and ill people, and the availability of images that show nurses tending the ostensibly sick (but somehow also glamorous), it is easy to believe that nurses do not see or touch blood, excrement or gore. Images of nurses soothingly caressing the foreheads of sick men (seldom sick women) still create potent fictions about the work of nurses.[1]

Within this particular fiction, nurses' interactions with sick bodies are of a soothing, maternal nature. Nurses, in this form of imagery, do not hurt or cause pain — their soothing touch makes it easier for the sick person, who is the recipient of these ministrations, to deal with pain. This makes the work of nurses with sick and injured bodies invisible. Yet is these types of bodies that nurses deal with on a day-to-day basis. The common experience of all types of nurses is of bodies in various states of injury, destruction, dysfunction, and/or illness.

Nurses use their own bodies as tools of their work and the patient/client's body is the site of that work. The body and its signs are read by nurses to determine need for specific nursing care. It is read again to determine if their attention to the person's needs has had the desired effect. The body signals, to its nurse readers, its dysfunction and its healing. To ignore these experiences is to continue the fictions about nurses and their work. This ignorance, ultimately a political action, denies both the realities of nurses' work and the opportunity of the public to enter into meaningful discourse about what it means to be sick, the social value of caring for others, or to challenge notions of bodily perfection. While making pictures of nurses working has personal benefits for me, it also provides opportunities for others. The pictures allow, even encourage, humans to look at the injured bodies of others without the chance of being rebuked for looking; images make voyeurs of us all. People can, at the same time, see the voyeurism inherent in nursing care, where a nurse can look, touch, expose and examine a person's body with impunity.

For people who are not nurses, my pictures offer the chance to look at nurses working with sick bodies and to contemplate and construct meanings for them. For nurses, the images can arouse thoughts and feelings about what it means to care for sick people. Nurse can also consider how, like photographs, the sick body provides them with evidence, tells stories and waits for them to bring meaning to it.

NOTES

1 See, for example, the photograph on the cover of the 1990s promotional pamphlet 'Nurses. We can't live without them', (New South Wales Health Department).

REFERENCES

Foucault M 1980 Michel Foucault: power/knowledge: selected interviews and other writings, 1972–1977. Harvester press, Brighton

Gilman S 1988 Disease and representation: images of illness from madness to AIDS. Cornell University Press, Ithaca

Hall S 1980 Encoding/decoding. In: Hall S, Lowe A, Hobson D (eds) Culture, media and language: working papers in cultural studies 1972–1979. Hutchinson, London

Rudisill 1982 On reading photographs. Journal of American Culture 5(3):1–15

Sekula A 1982 On the invention of photographic meaning. In: Burgin V (ed) Thinking photography. Macmillan, London

Sontag S 1977 Illness as metaphor. Vintage Books, New York

Sontag S 1979 On photography. Straus and Giroux, London

Tagg J 1988 The burden of representation. Essays on photographies and histories. Macmillan, London

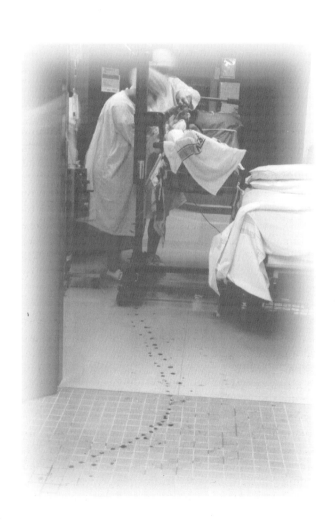

3

The body as text and the body as living flesh

Metaphors of the body and nursing in postmodernity

Judith Parker

Introduction

Nurses work closely with other people's bodies and the body is therefore a central concern in nursing practice. Until recently, study of the body in nursing has been undertaken almost exclusively within the scientific discourse of modern medicine. Here the body has been constituted as an object of nature and understood metaphorically as a machine. Understandings about the body, and indeed of the nature of nursing, have therefore been dominated by medicine, modernity and the machine metaphor. Lately, however, some critiques have emerged from within science and social and cultural theory that raise questions about the modernist notions within which both the body and nursing have been understood. These critiques can be loosely drawn together under the umbrella term of postmodernity.

Ways of thinking that are emerging in postmodernity enable us to think of bodies as texts. Bodies are constituted and produced by various historical and cultural markings upon the body. Bodies vary across time and space and are formed through historical and cultural patterns of thought and action, i.e. through discursive formations. These formations are linked to power. For example, observation of bodies as portrayed in European paintings over time helps us to understand that the constitution of the body as a child is a relatively recent phenomenon. The body as a child is linked to the historical and political factors surrounding industrialisation and the emergence of compulsory schooling. The child, it would seem, is a product of modernity. However, it is now becoming clear that we live in the postmodern terrain of global information systems and rapidly changing patterns of work. In this chapter the body as text is a metaphoric way of understanding how information technology, biotechnology and the rationalising processes inherent within emerging health structures are helping to constitute both the body and nursing in postmodernity.

The body as living flesh, by contrast, evokes notions of the vulnerability, contingency and eventual decrepitude of embodiment. It therefore invites an attitude of recognition of and respect for our mutual frailties as embodied beings. As nurses we are only too well aware that touching a person in the context of the provision of nursing care can be a source of profound comfort. However we also know that touch can be felt as an invasion which reduces a person's sense of being to that of an object or a thing, particularly when one is feeling vulnerable. What is highlighted here is the fragility of body boundaries and the consolation or violation that can be felt at the interpenetrating margins of bodies. The body as living flesh is a metaphoric way of understanding the spaces between the discursive imprints upon the body. It is a way of understanding the atextual body. The body as living flesh is an embodied space from which creativity and new understandings can emerge.

This chapter approaches the metaphoric constitution of the body in nursing as text and as living flesh within a broader discussion of modernity and postmodernity generally. I want to pay heed to what I think of as three mutually constitutive qualities of human life and cultural production: the qualities of time, space and knowledge. I will consider some aspects of the constitution of these qualities within modernity and postmodernity. Because of their mutually constitutive nature, consideration of each quality requires some discussion of the others.

I also want to consider the constitution of the body/subject and nursing in light of these qualities. Specifically, I want to consider the body/subject in relation to death, colonisation and knowledge, and nursing in relation to time, colonisation and work. It is within this context that I will begin to explore some issues surrounding the body as text and as living flesh. Throughout the chapter, I am suggesting that in postmodernity both nursing and the body are characterised by collapsing hierarchies and polarities with the emergence of heterogeneities, pluralities and a concern with surfaces. However, I am also suggesting that within the ambiguous and incommensurate spaces created by the falling away of these divisions, new understandings about the body and nursing can emerge.

The constitution of time

With the French Enlightenment there arose a notion of the modern which delineates the philosophy and values of the 'age of reason' and concomitant notions of growth and progress linked to individual and social betterment through the use of reason. This idea of the modern has provided a philosophy and rationale for the development of both the socialist and liberal democratic societies that have arisen in Europe, in Britain and in many of the countries they colonised. It has underpinned the emergence of modern forms of institutions, such as medicine and law, and the modern structure of systems of health care and social regulation which have developed in the public domain. It has provided the principles that have supported the policies of colonialism and expansionism on a global scale which occurred with the emergence of industrialisation and the application of scientific principles to the workplace. It has provided the rationale for the emergence of the modern hospital and for modern professional nursing. Within this context the person has been understood in dualistic terms, with the body constituted as an object of medical scientific investigation and treatment.

The term 'postmodernity' suggests that it is somehow 'after modernity'. But postmodernity is not an historical era which follows the era of modernity. Postmodernity coexists with modernity. An understanding of what it means to be 'after' modernity in the postmodern sense requires some consideration of the modern. Here I am drawing upon the work of Habermas who points out that the term 'modern' has been around since the fifth century. He notes that '[w]ith varying content, the term "modern" again and again expresses the consciousness of an epoch that relates itself to the past of antiquity, in order to view itself as the result of a transition from the old to the new' (Habermas 1983:3). The modern was defined in relation to the authority of the past.

What is of particular importance to an understanding of the relationship between modernity and postmodernity, is the significant change in ideas about the modern that took place within the context of the ideals of the French Enlightenment. Instead of looking back to the authority of the past to define the modern, there emerged a belief, inspired by modern science, 'in the infinite progress of knowledge and in the infinite advance towards social and moral betterment' (Habermas 1983:4). Modernity thus came to be defined in terms of progress and development brought about by the use of reason and through advances in science and technology. Above all, modernity is concerned with notions of a better future.

This changed understanding of the modern and the idea of futurity, associated with belief in the progress of knowledge, took place in the context of the rise of the middle class in Europe. This era also saw the emergence of the autonomous (male) individual, or self, with an identity formed through individual achievements arising out of projects directed towards advancing the visions of modernity. This is in contrast to the identities which were formed through recreating the past, through being ascribed a particular status, usually inherited, as occurred in feudal societies. In modernity an individual achieving self emerged which was linked to a class structure in society and oriented to the future rather than the past. This is not to say that with modernity the premodern time orientation lapsed. Rather, the time orientation of modernity coexisted alongside the premodern.

Heller and Feher (1988) point out that to be postmodern is to be after the 'grand narrative', i.e. after the sacred story of 'the project of Europe' with its mythological and symbolic claims about the universality and unashamed superiority of European culture. Postmodernity can then be thought of as 'after modernity' in the sense of 'after' loss of belief in a future oriented way of understanding social reality; a future that has associated with it belief in the possibility of the implementation of the modernist vision, belief in the transcendent power of science and rationality and belief in the infinite progress of knowledge and development. Postmodernity implies a collapse in belief in the European colonising impulses and activities of modernity.

In modernity, time came to be conceived of in dualistic terms, so that time consciousness was understood to comprise the two dimensions, inner time and outer time. Bergson (1965) used the term duration *(dureé)* to describe immediately perceived inner time. He described it as 'the very fluidity of our inner life', an 'uninterrupted transition, multiplicity without divisibility and succession without separation'. Outer time, by contrast, gives form to the content of inner time. Outer time is socially constructed temporality. It frames and gives shape to inner time. In modernity this outer time is quantified, linear and historicised time. In modernity, time has been experienced diachronically as an inner experience within the context of cultural notions of linearity and historical development. Temporality has thus been conceived of in terms of the depth of its dual dimensions.

In postmodernity, these inner/outer distinctions collapse so that time is experienced synchronically. Consequently, there is a loss of depth in the experience of time as the form and content of time, the inner and outer dimensions, interpenetrate each other. This results in a feeling of everything happening at once, a flattened sense of the presentness of time, rather than as a time ordered sequence within history. The structuring of history into a linear story of progress and futurity has collapsed. This is what is meant when postmodernity is described as posthistory. Heller and Feher (1988) suggest that what is new about postmodernity is the novel historical consciousness that has emerged. Those in postmodernity have a sense of being permanently in the present and at the same time after it. Heller and Feher claim that in postmodernity the present has been appropriated more profoundly than ever before.

The self in postmodernity is thus constituted in relation to neither the past, nor the future; neither to a feudal premodern identity constituted through recreating the past nor to an individual class based identity constituted through futurity and the hope of implementing the modernist vision. Postmodernity suggests an orientation to a present with neither a glorious mythological past nor a visionary future. It means being lodged uneasily in a permanent present with a collapsed sense of time, without beginning and without end, without history or hope. The present is the only eternity.

However, it is important to understand, as Heller and Feher (1988:1) point out, those who 'dwell in postmodernity...live among moderns as well as premoderns', and that in postmodernity it is possible to develop a critical distance from the immediacy of presentness. Postmodernity is a temporality of presentness among a plurality of other temporalities. However it is a significant temporality of this age in its constitution as a flattened sense of presentness and simultaneity.

I now want to consider some implications of the changing constitution of time in postmodernity, first in relation to the idea of death and then in relation to nursing work.

The body/subject and death

In modernity, subjectivity came to be understood as separate from both the body and the external world. The self which was linked to the disembodied mind was conceived of as an essence. It was continuous over time and space, and had control over the body. This self was regarded as autonomous, free and independent. Thus self-identity was not so immediately and materially tied to physical and spatial boundaries, which, it was believed, could be transcended. It seems that in this context the body came to be distrusted and conceived of as a source of threat. This is not surprising given the future orientation of modernity, and its links to projects of mastery through achievements of individuals striving to implement its futuristic visions. The contingent nature of the body can constrain, limit, subvert and prohibit the projects of the striving subject. It has the capacity to disrupt projects directed to the future. Bodily decrepitude can interfere with the plans and projects of the subject; death has the power to destroy them. In this sense the body has been a dark shadow over the glorious visions of modernity, uneasily threatening to undermine its projects.

Philosopher and physician Drew Leder (1992) has claimed that medicine in modernity is 'profoundly Cartesian in spirit'. By this he means that it is fundamentally concerned with gaining mastery over the threat of death posed by the mortal body. With the emergence of science and medicine the body came to be conceived of as part of nature and paradoxically understood metaphorically as a machine, as an object which could be repaired if parts broke down. Scientific theory could offer the hope of overcoming the travails of disease and suffering, and modern medicine has sought to provide investigations and therapies aimed at managing the uncertainties and vulnerabilities of perishable embodied existence. It is not surprising that belief in the power of medicine to prevent death has emerged so strongly in modernity and that underlying the projects of modernity there is a prevailing anxiety about death. Indeed Freud, who wrote at the height of the universalising impulses of modernity posited a death instinct.

Recently a British medical practitioner involved in the hospice movement in that country for many years stated: 'the Christian foundation for hospice work...is already attenuated in a society not embarrassed by sex or death now, but immediately ill at ease with any mention of God or spiritual distress' (Wilkes 1994:4). A postmodern reading of this statement might suggest that the Cartesian death anxiety has been assuaged in the context of the collapse of time and the breakdown of belief in the narratives of progress and achievement of modernity. In a sensibility characterised by an orientation to presentness rather than to futurity, death is not such a pressing concern.

Time and nursing work

While death anxiety may have been a major force driving the investigative and therapeutic endeavours of modern medicine, most nurses working within medically dominated contexts have not had such a single-minded commitment to the achievement of future oriented curative goals. A commonplace of nursing is that nurses are witness to the suffering of patients in a way that doctors are not. In concentrating on the nursing measures of care and comfort they are therefore more attuned to immediacy, and to the demands of the moment. They are less anxious about death and much more concerned with the alleviation of suffering. Many of the conflicts that have arisen between doctors and nurses within the hospital context can be described in terms of the oppositions between care and cure. These can be understood as conflicting temporalities, one directed to the present time, the other directed towards the future. These can also be understood as competing ideologies of health care.

Conflicts that have arisen between doctors and nurses have occurred especially in contexts dominated by the imperatives of curative medicine which have tended to marginalise and silence the nursing voice (Parker & Gardner 1992). Here doctors have been positioned as the powerful striving subjects of modernity preventing death, while nurses have been positioned as the nurturant objects of nature subserviently complicit in medical curative projects while offering comfort measures to the patients in their care. They have thus been positioned between the doctor and the patient, understanding of both. As Trinh Minh-Ha (1992) points out, 'dominated and marginalized people have been socialized to see always more than their own point of view.'

To the extent that there is a weakening of the modernist temporality directed towards the future, there is opportunity for the nursing voice that articulates the concerns of the moment to be heard. However, contemporary health care is in the throes of significant change. The nurse is now in the space where everything is happening at once, attuned to the positionings and imperatives of various temporalities. These include not only those of the doctor and the patient, but also those of the economically driven demands for shorter length of stay and increased throughput of patients. In trying to meet competing and possibly incommensurate demands, the nurse may well locate him or herself in the ambiguous spaces between the competing temporalities. This idea will be developed further in a consideration of the constitution of space.

The constitution of space

The Australia of modernity emerged out of the unashamed cultural supremacy of the colonising impulses inherent within the notions of Europe and Empire. There was a time when Australian children of modernity learned in school about the 'all red route' traversed by ships sailing around the world. Maps had marked upon them in red the routes taken which ensured ships berthed only at ports that were part of the British Empire. Children learned that 'the sun never set on the British Empire'. The process of colonisation was sustained by a grand story of expanding time and space and it was inspired by the visions of infinite development and betterment of all, including those unfortunate enough not to be European (or more specifically in the Australian context, British). This colonising process dichotomised people into the colonisers and the colonised. The colonisers were those who identified with the universalising claims of the endeavours of modernity. The colonised were seen as the 'other', as everything the colonisers were not. The colonised became objects of study, definition and redefinition (Hartsock 1990:61).

In postmodernity, writers (e.g. Bhabha 1994) have identified a shift from a European class based and a Eurocentric colonising/colonised sense of space to a disoriented presence between a plurality of heterogeneous spaces. This shift is linked to both the increasing pluralisation of cultures which has occurred within the West and to the collapse of the colonial system. Postmodernity is thus characterised by a shift away from belief in the pre-eminence of Europe (in the Australian context, that of Britain) with its modernist colonising gaze. The effect has been a shift away from the historical time consciousness of modernity and belief in its universalising projects. A plurality of cultures has emerged with a heterogeneity of temporalities, constituted in the context of a range of various local and small narratives (e.g. cultural, religious, ethnic).

Heller and Feher's (1988) work helps in understanding how the pluralisation of western cultures that has taken place over the last fifty years has contributed to the radical weakening of the European project of modernity. They describe three consecutive cultural generations or waves that have occurred in the West since the Second World War. Each, they say, 'continues the pluralization of the cultural universe in modernity as well as the destruction of class cultures' (p.136). They suggest that these waves have been vehicles of profound change in the patterns of everyday life in western culture. They describe them as the existentialist, the alienation and the postmodernist generations.

The existential wave was 'the first in a series of the most striking phenomena of western history in the second half of the twentieth century' (Heller & Feher 1988:137). The postwar existentialist generation involved a rebellion of subjectivity. Young people were intent on breaking free, on practising their freedom within the constraints that limited them. The alienation generation of the 1960s, by contrast, was 'the dusk of subjectivity and freedom' and through an outgrowth of despair, liberation movements were born. The postmodern generation has emerged in the 1980s and it is neither conservative, revolutionary or progressive. It is a wave 'of boundless pluralism' in which all kinds of things are possible and one in which 'anything goes'.

The collapse of the colonial system is also a significant aspect of postmodernity. Owens (1993) claims that Ricoeur's recognition that 'the discovery of the plurality of cultures is never a harmless experience, is perhaps the most eloquent testimony to the end of Western sovereignty'. Owens highlights the coexistence of different cultures as a characteristic of a postmodern age. He cites Ricoeur's words: 'Suddenly it becomes possible that there are just *others*, that we ourselves are an "other" among others.' What is at stake then, Owens argues, 'is not only the hegemony of Western culture, but also (our sense of) our identity as a culture'. For a European to arrive at this understanding is to have his or her belief in the universality and superiority of western culture radically disturbed. This is a profoundly disrupting experience. Heller and Feher (1988) make the point that the cultural and political campaign *against* ethnocentrism has in fact been a major campaign *for* postmodernity.

Bhabha (1994:1) takes this understanding further in the context of postcoloniality. He claims that '[o]ur existence today is marked by a tenebrous sense of survival, living on the border lines of the present, for which there seems to be no proper name other than the current and controversial shiftiness of the prefix "post"'. He makes the point that a border or boundary is not where something stops. It is not a mark of closure. Rather a border, as Heidegger (in Bhabha 1994:1) noted, 'is that from which something begins its presencing'. Thus the spatiality of postmodernity is characterised as being present (i.e. here, now) at the edge of the beyond, a presence in an in–between space which is distinguished by 'a sense of disorientation, a disturbance of direction'.

It is worth reiterating that postmodernity is characterised by plurality and heterogeneity. Thus, it would seem that the temporality and spatiality of modernity, which projects a progressive and spatially expanding future and which turns its back on the past becomes one among other spatiotemporal realities. However this is a relativist position which implies some sort of 'level playing field' within which multiple temporalities and spatialities are played out. It fails to take into account power relations and the rationalising and colonising imperatives of late modernity. These ideas will be taken up in the discussion to follow.

I now want to consider some of the implications of the changing constitution of space in postmodernity. Specifically, I want to consider implications for the body/subject and nursing, first in relation to the idea of the colonised body and then in relation to colonisation and nursing.

The colonised body

In the premodern era, the body was part of the sacred realm. However, in modernity the body has become naturalised and it has come to be conceived of as an object or thing within the natural world. In becoming secularised and objectified it has come to be understood as a machine and opened up to scrutiny and scientific investigation. It has been studied as a material causal entity, a physically determined object of scientific investigation and treatment. In becoming a thing it has separated from the essential person. In this way it has become an 'other' available to the colonising impulses of modernity.

In modernity the body has become, metaphorically, a territory to be explored and conquered through the activities of medical expansionism, a continent to be opened up, divided and shared among specialties and sub-specialties. This is what is meant by the colonisation of the body by medicine. The objectifying tendencies inherent in therapeutic endeavours and the Cartesian anxiety about death can be seen as powerfully constitutive of the modernist vision to be achieved through the investigative and therapeutic endeavours of modern medicine.

Through this process the body has become commodified and it also has become an object providing commercial advantage to its colonisers. Illich (1986) has pointed out that the image of the body as an object of medical colonisation was at its most powerful and far reaching in the 1950s and 1960s.

He suggests that by '[a]round the middle of this century, the medical establishment reached an unprecedented influence over the social construction of bodies... We experienced a special moment of history, when one agency, namely medicine, reached toward a monopoly over the social construction of bodily reality'. In this context it is not surprising that the body has emerged as a medical commodity.

This progressive medicalisation of the body can be understood as having occurred contemporaneously with the colonisation and commodification that occurred in the context of European global expansionism. However, like colonisation, and no doubt subject to the same destabilising forces which have affected modernity generally, the monopoly over the body held by medicine began to wane. By the 1980s, as Illich points out, the medical hegemony over the body had weakened considerably and practices of commodification of the body were being shared with other agents. These include not only complementary therapists and health and fitness personnel, for example, working on the bodies of others, but also individuals conceiving of themselves as producers of their bodies, engaged in the project of body shaping and forming.

With an attenuation of death anxiety and a greater orientation to the present, wherein lifestyles are constituted through bodies (aesthetic, fashion, sporting, shaping), the body is becoming a highly contested site for colonising and commodification by many different cultures and practices. In this sense the colonised body of postmodernity is a body of multiplicities and surfaces, amenable to a plurality of practices, to recycling rather that to maturation and decline.

The natural body of modernity was a body of depths comprising outer and inner dimensions. It was a finite body with a future that would end in death. The task of medicine was to plumb its depths and bring its secrets to light in pursuit of preventing death. However, developments in what has come to be called postmodern medicine point to an understanding of the body which is markedly different from that constituted within modern medicine. Thus the primacy and ubiquity of the modernist and scientific understandings of the body are being challenged from within science itself.

Writers such as Levin and Solomon (1990), for example, point out that late modern medicine has studied the invisible interiority of the flesh so deeply that the old boundaries articulating the body in terms of an external and internal reality no longer make sense. They describe how it is no longer appropriate to draw distinctions between body and mind, because it now can be demonstrated that we understand the world through our muscles, tendons and joints and thus meaning can no longer be thought of as a function of the disembodied mind. Psychoneuroimmunological medicine demonstrates that distinctions cannot be drawn between the individual and the environment and thus the distinctions drawn in modernity between subject and object collapse. In postmodern medicine, the body has come to be thought of metaphorically as a communication field, as a text which can be read by advanced technology.

Haraway (1990) argues that the biomedical, biotechnical body is a complex meaning producing field in which disease is now being understood as a sub species of information malfunction or communications pathology. As Illich (1986) has noted, this age may bring forth 'people who experience themselves as contributors to a complex computer program and...see themselves as part of the text'. It is this flattened, spatialised, denaturalised body that I am referring to metaphorically as the body as text. Levin and Solomon (1990) make the point that medicine now can, for the first time, formulate very specific correlations between the patient's bodily experienced meanings and the conditions and states of the medical body, i.e. the body which features in the research and clinical practice of medicine. Thus the body as text can be read not only by the medical practitioner, but also by those patients who are willing to train themselves to the prescribed level of body awareness.

This opens up new opportunities for nursing. For example, nurses are developing therapeutic and educative roles in the context of psycho-neuroimmunological medicine. These aim to facilitate people's increasing embodied awareness and the textual expression of precisely distinguished bodily meanings. This is likely to be very popular in nursing as it will provide nurses with a range of therapeutic technologies they can practise within a value system of empowerment of the client. An example is therapeutic touch, which until recently has been marginal in health care because no scientific rationale could be provided (Quinn & Strelkauskas 1993).

Ingham (1989), in a review of the nursing literature on touch, concluded that further research should be undertaken to explore nurses' awareness and use of touch. One can anticipate a flourishing of technologies of touch as this type of research is translated into practice. Studies involving explorations of body listening are also being reported in the literature (e.g. Price 1993) and alternative, complementary and holistic health therapies such as shiatsu and aroma therapy, which can also be understood as technologies facilitating body awareness, are being incorporated into mainstream nursing. One could envisage these being reframed so as to be made consistent with the imperatives of psychoneuroimmunological medicine.

I have identified a number of colonised bodies which have been inscribed by the marks of colonising agents. These include the anatomical body, which can be understood as a political body inscribed by the discourses of modern medicine and indeed modern western culture. This is the body of modernity fuelled by anxiety about death. There are the commodified bodies of our lifestyle oriented and market driven postmodern popular culture and the bodies colonised by various groups who set themselves up as body experts purveying a range of body therapeutics. There is the body of late modern medicine colonised by biotechnology and advanced communication systems. Each of these indicates how bodies are inscribed or marked and how they serve as signifiers or texts which can be read by others.

With the denaturalisation of the body, understandings about mind and subjectivity have also changed. In postmodernity, subjectivity is no longer thought of as residing in the disembodied mind, separated from the external world of objects. Indeed, modernist notions of the self are being increasingly called into question from many sources. Feminists, for example, have claimed that the notion of personhood inherent in this self is male and that it therefore does not provide a satisfactory account of the embodied sense of self of women's experience. Social theorists, historians and anthropologists have argued that the notions of an isolated consciousness and an essential self are problematic in light of historical and cultural relativities. Linguists have deconstructed the division between the conceptual signifier and the material/expressive signified, which was based on a mind/body dichotomy. This has resulted in a shift away from a concern with consciousness, that is with mind, to an emphasis on language which is performative rather than denotative. Here language is not thought of as representing reality, but rather as 'a discursive practice that enacts or produces that which it names' (Butler 1993:13). Other social theorists and critics of modernity have attempted to undermine or offer resistance to the projects which flowed from modernist ideas about the autonomy and radical freedom of the subject.

Under the influence of poststructural thought, subjectivity is now being conceived of as decentred and constituted within the various discourses which bring phenomena into being. In postmodernity there have been attempts to refocus on corporeality in accounts of subjectivity. As Grosz (1994:vii) states: 'All the effects of depth and interiority can be explained in terms of the inscriptions and transformations of the subject's corporeal surface'. She claims that various cultural and historical inscriptions 'quite literally constitute bodies and help to produce them as such'. These constitutions of the body/subject involve a shift away from an understanding of the body as a mechanistic, determinate object controlled by a decorporealised self, to a concern with surfaces and a shifting, changing subjectivity constituted by discourses.

Colonisation and nursing

Nursing, like the body, can be thought of as having been colonised by the objectifying and rationalising impulses of modern medicine within the context of the institutional structures of the health system of modernity. I am arguing here that nursing continues to be colonised in the context of imperatives of postmodern science and advanced communication technologies. These bring with them new colonising forms. In postmodernity, as Haraway (1990) points out, prior means of control and repression have given way to new forms. She says: 'Dominations no longer work through medicalization and normalization, but through networking, communication redesign and stress management'.

Other imperatives of postmodernity are also contributing to changes in nursing. Of significance here are the changes taking place in the spatial organisation of nursing. The institutional health structures of modernity were hierarchical, with boundaries clearly delineated by gradings of seniority, discrete functional units and geographically discrete units of care. So called 'post institutional' structures by contrast are more flattened with boundaries formed at local levels in the provision of 'seamless' continuity of care.

The structure and organisation of nursing work is changing dramatically as old hierarchies and boundaries break down and new health care structures emerge. The information systems which supported separate and specific functional units have given way to those using integrated data bases. The new structures are dominated by the imperatives of advanced communication technologies and the quantifying impulses of economic rationalism. In the spatialisation of health structures there has been a spatialisation of nursing so that it has come to be constituted as a unit of information in the costing of services.

In this context, a nurse at work may find him or herself positioned between competing spatiotemporalities and effectively they are caught between future oriented curative medical goals and the patient's immediate situation. They may find themselves caught between medical demands for patient compliance and their assessment that the patient has different priorities. They may feel disquiet at the subtler forms of rationality at work within processes that allow little space for difference as patients' episodes of hospitalisation are managed through costed care plans. They may find themselves caught between demands for reductions in the quantified time of care episodes and the demands associated with nursing work to be completed over the timespan of a shift. They may feel caught between the demands stemming from the embodied temporality of endurance experienced by some patients in the ongoing immediacy of pain and suffering and the colonised self gaze of other patients less immersed in the immediacies of bodily insistence.

The temporality constituted by a nurse on a particular shift will be a function of a complex interplay of factors to do with the nurse's own history and disposition, his or her sense of colonisation, the imperatives of the work situation and any number of fortuitous contingencies. Over the duration of a period on duty, the nurse is positioned between sets of contesting temporalities constituted by medical treatment regimens, institutional requirements for productivity and increased throughput with measurable outcomes, the pressingness of the patient's needs and the designated nursing work load for the rostered shift.

In this context a number of temporalities will intersect to create an uneasy space. This strikes me as being not unlike the description of the space 'of disorientation, a disturbance of direction'. Trinh Minh-Ha (1992), who writes in the context of the complex reality of postcoloniality, argues that it is vital for dominated and marginalised people to recognise the ambiguity of their 'in-between' location and draw upon this understanding of incommensurabilities to 'assume one's radical "impurity" and...recognise the necessity of speaking from a hybrid place, hence of saying at least two, three things at a time'. It seems to me that there are many parallels here for nurses in the complex terrains of 'post institutional' health care. The nurse in this sense is hybrid, able to speak the voices of medicine nursing, institution and patient. Rather than being confused and disoriented by this multivocality, the nurse can assume a position 'in between'. It is from this place that new understandings and previously hidden dimensions of nursing may emerge. It is the space 'in-between' that I am describing in terms of the metaphor of the body as living flesh.

The cultural production of knowledge

I now want to shift to an examination of changing understandings about the cultural production of knowledge in postmodernity. These have resulted in a blurring of boundaries between previously discrete forms of knowledge. They also challenge notions of the possibility of the production of objective knowledge and emphasise the emergence of a proliferation of competing truth claims.,I will start by returning again to the work of Habermas.

In delineating aspects of what he describes as the project of modernity, Habermas (1983) draws upon Weber's characterisation of cultural modernity. He identifies this project as being formulated, consistent with Enlightenment ideals, in terms of efforts to develop the separate spheres of 'objective science, universal morality and law, and autonomous art according to their inner logic'. This logic was understood as the form of rationality which was intrinsic to each sphere; cognitive — instrumental for science, moral — practical for morality, and aesthetic — expressive for art. A significant aim of the project of modernity was to utilise this 'accumulation of specialised culture for the enrichment of everyday life' (Habermas 1983:9).

Habermas points out, however, that this process of cultural rationalisation resulted in the three domains of culture becoming quite separate, not only from each other, but also from the everyday life-world. They were organised into autonomous cultural professions which were controlled by specialised experts. As a consequence, scientific discourse, theories of morality and jurisprudence, and the production and criticism of art became the property of specialists within these autonomous spheres. This led to the separation of these spheres from the 'hermeneutics of everyday communication' (1983:9). Contrary to the dreams of the Enlightenment philosophers, there emerged a split between the esoteric, specialised culture of the experts and professionals and the commonplace culture of everyday life.

This reading of Habermas helps us to understand postmodernity as a breaking down or blurring of and rendering ambiguous the boundaries between the previously autonomous spheres of specialised knowledge in modernity. What is at stake here is the authority and power of the culture of professional expertise which surrounded the construction of truth (science), virtue (law and ethics), and beauty (art). The breaking down of these barriers has been taking place in the context of challenges being mounted, by contemporary cultural and feminist scholars and others, particularly to the claims made for these spheres of knowledge that they are based in a logic of rationality.

The questioning of modernist notions of the primacy of rationality in the construction of knowledge, together with the blurring or breaking down of previously clearly delineated boundaries between spheres of knowledge has been described as 'a crisis of cultural authority, specifically of the authority vested in Western European culture and its institutions' Owens (1983). Feminist critiques of and challenges to the patriarchal assumptions and understandings central to the various spheres of knowledge, as well as to everyday life, have contributed to this crisis.

Knowledge production in modernity has been based on a belief that the task of knowledge was to build an adequate representation of things (Benhabib 1990). This was done through developing concepts and conceptual frameworks to represent experience. However, these schema tend to homogenise and render static the complex heterogeneity and fluidity of experience. They become stultifying edifices which privilege and hold fast certain aspects of experience while hiding, diminishing or ignoring others. They serve as instruments of colonisation and are maintained through authority, power and vested interests. The nursing theories which emerged in the 1960s and 1970s can certainly be understood in this way.

Critiques of this form of knowledge production have been mounted on several fronts. Various truth claims of science have been deconstructed and hence contested through demonstrating that their claims to universality are historically specific. In responding to the universalising 'mastery' techniques of modernity, postmodernists and feminists seek to deconstruct the homogenising concepts of modernity and patriarchy so as to open up their closed systems to the heterogeneity of experience. This has resulted in a proliferation of competing knowledge claims by various groups. Benhabib (1990) points out that the breakdown in the rigidity of modernist knowledge production and the eclecticism and fluidity flowing from the dissolution of the episteme of representation has resulted in a 'dazzling play of surfaces' as knowledge is constructed from a variety of sources.

In this context it is not surprising that postmodern knowledge has come to be thought of as inextricably linked to power (Foucault 1980). Knowledge is only made possible and is only able to function through regimes of power. But at the same time, as forms of knowledge transform so power is transformed. However, as Lyotard (1984) has stated '[p]ostmodern knowledge is not simply an instrument of power. It refines our sensitivity to differences and increases our tolerance of incommensurability'.

Knowledge and the body

The preceding analysis helps us to understand that in modernity the body has been constituted within the scientific domain of knowledge and maintained through the authority of the disciplinary power of modern medicine. This has meant that other ways of thinking about the body have been marginalised or silenced. However, critiques of the dichotomies of modernity formulated by feminist and cultural theorists have opened up spaces for understanding the body in a variety of ways. There is now a plethora of competing and sometimes incommensurate knowledges of the body linked to various regimes of power, for example, those linked to various cultural and spiritual body practices and those promulgated by the power of the media and advertising. Some of these are at play in the complex terrains of 'post institutional' health care where bodies are nursed.

Postmodern knowledge helps us to understand how we can think of bodies generally as texts. The particular body as text that I am interested in is the body being constituted by the discourses of postmodern medicine and 'post institutional' health care structures. Some of the implications for the constitution and regulation of this body, which stem from understandings about advanced technologies and communication systems, are now being made clear. Here the body as text is a metaphorical means of grasping the subtle yet powerful sets of rationalising processes at work within our health care system.

The body as text does not suggest a radical break or rupture from the colonising imperatives of modernity. Rather, it indicates a continuity of these processes of domination now being driven particularly by the forces of economic rationalism. In postulating the body as living flesh, I am endeavouring to find a means of imagining ways of resisting the imperatives of these rationalising forces. Specifically I am describing the body in this way as a metaphor for the spaces between the text, as a way of imagining the pretextual or atextual body. The body as living flesh is a metaphorical way of creating space for an exploration of the betweenness of bodies in nursing. It may include an exploration of nurses' experience of bodies with overflowing boundaries (see Wiltshire & Parker 1996).

The notion of the body as living flesh has its origins in the work of Merleau-Ponty (1962) who conceived of the body as neither a mechanical thing nor as a flattened text or communication field. As Grosz (1994:90) points out, for Merleau-Ponty, 'the body is fundamentally linked to representations of spatiality and temporality'. She quotes Merleau-Ponty: 'Our body is not in space like things; it inhabits or haunts space'.

While the body is a reference point for our spatiality, it is not an object viewed in a distant way by an observing subject. We have a different relationship with our body than we have to other objects. Drew Leder (1992) in drawing upon Merleau-Ponty, points out that the body is never first an object in the world, but the very medium by which our body comes into being. Our body mediates the world for us, is the medium for our appropriation of the world and is our anchorage in the world.

In his last work Merleau-Ponty (1968) describes the body as opening up the sense of everything there is, Being, which is fleshy. He describes Being in terms of the 'constant chiasm', the crisscrossing of 'seer and seen, the invisible and the visible, consciousness and object, the physical order and the vital order, the touching hand and the touched' (cited in Park 1983). Embodiment is understood as an interfolding of being and world. This understanding of the body thus breaks down the Cartesian binary division between body and mind. The metaphor of flesh implicates nature and embodiment as living and interconnected. But this is not an organismic model in which humanness is understood simply as part of the interconnectedness of nature. Merleau-Ponty refers to the notion of the intertwined nature of language and corporeality in the lived body.

Grosz (1994) points out that Merleau-Ponty's work 'in ways that surprisingly anticipate Derrida's supplementary readings of dichotomous polarizations, attempts to take up and utilize the space in between, the "no man's land" or gulf separating oppositional terms' (p.94). She goes on to make the point that his 'understanding of the constructed, synthetic nature of experience, its simultaneously active and passive functioning, its role in both the inscription and subversion of sociopolitical values, provides a crucial confirmation of many feminists' unspoken assumptions regarding women's experiences' (p.95).

The notion of the body as living flesh is not set up as a model of the body in opposition to the body as text. Rather, it is a metaphor for the space between discursive formations which render homogeneous the complexity and diversity of embodied experiences. The body as living flesh is a space of resistance, a space apart from rationalising and totalising processes, a space that permits the emergence of new understandings.

It evokes notions of the body/subject and the world in which body/subjects are constituted in terms of vulnerability, frailty and contingency. It is a metaphor which captures the in-between spaces where nursing is located. A nursing practice constituted, guided and sustained by this metaphor is unlikely to be pulled unreflectively by the imperatives of cybernetics, biotechnologies and the 'informatics of domination'. There is continuity between modernity's projects of mastery and the biotechnical and communication projects of postmodernity. Both suggest the hubris of human desire. The body as living flesh is a lesson in humility and compassion which sharpens our sense of the contingency of our endeavours yet which also gives us space to explore ambiguities and incommensurabilities and to act cautiously, reflectively and with understandings stemming from experience.

Knowledge and nursing work

Habermas' analysis of modernity helps us to see that the modern hospital has been structured in terms of scientific principles, with a division of labour based on areas of specialised knowledge with clear differentiation between the cultural domains of expert knowledge and that of everyday life. Within this context modern professional nursing emerges as a fundamentally ambiguous activity. Since it arose in the late nineteenth century it has been characterised by two major sets of tensions. One of these breached the public/private divisions which emerged with the modernist era, while the other breached the division between the everyday and the specialised cultural domains. Nursing was located in the public realm with a brief to undertake intimate and personal tasks normally performed within the private realm of the family. Additionally, as an occupation dealing with mundane matters of comfort and care, it breached the divisions between the culture of everyday life and that of the specialised, 'high' culture of science and medicine in daring to pursue professional legitimacy.

In nursing there has been a tension between the private and the public sphere which has been generated in relation to nurses' (public) role in dealing with the (private) body (Lawler 1991). This has been managed historically in two (ambiguously interrelated) ways, both of which involve the portrayal of the nurse as female. Both evoke positive images of the nurse and both place strong sanctions on nurses to conform to these positive images. One has been the invocation of the nurse as an angel of mercy, etherealised and linked to the historic role of the Church. Here the nurse touches the body reverently as in a Christian laying on of hands and thereby makes the body sacred and takes both nurse and patient out of the secular domain. The other has been the portrayal of the nurse as a maternal figure, desexualised through elevation in status to wife (of the doctor) and mother (of the patient) in the medically controlled hospital family. Here the nurse touches the body as an idealised mother touches the body of a child, nurturantly, skilfully and with authority.

Both portrayals mask the complex ambiguities at the core of nursing operations that have remained submerged in modernity.

A postmodern analysis of nursing in relation to the divisions which arose in modernity helps us to think about nurses as positioned indeterminately between a number of normatively bounded entities within health care. They are situated at the interface of therapeutic intervention and expressive connection; between doing for and being with. They work at the overlapping, interpenetrating margins between professional constraint and personal intimacy. They trouble the borders of bodily eruption/disruption and bodily hygiene and order. They are located precariously between the world of the doctor and the patient. As a consequence of these equivocal locations, nurses work on a daily basis in a context of uncertainty, paradox and incommensurability. The body as living flesh is a metaphor for exploring the space between these dichotomous polarisations in nursing.

The boundaries surrounding the cultural production of knowledge have been very clearly delineated in modernity. Thus those dimensions of nursing knowledge and knowledge of the body, which reside in the borderlands between a range of discrete fields, have been rendered silent. Critiques of various aspects of modernity are helping to open spaces for nursing inquiry. These include critiques stemming from the history and philosophy of science, feminist critiques of the patriarchal nature of science, methodological critiques of the abstracted, decontextualised nature of scientific method applied to the social world, critiques of modernist ethical schemes and emerging understandings about the relationships between art and everyday activities. Nurses who dwell in postmodernity can thus draw upon these critiques in exploring the indeterminate sphere of the borderlands to articulate nursing voices of the in-between.

Concluding thoughts

The body as text is a metaphor which captures the changing constitution of the body in postmodernity. The constitutive metaphor for the body in the industrial age of modernity was a machine. Here the body was conceived of as a natural three dimensional object. The metaphor of text captures the flattened sense of the postmodern age and its communicative imperatives. It indicates the power of discourses to create, control and constrain phenomena. In this sense everything is a text. I have used the metaphor of the body as text as a way of understanding the constitution of the body within the rationalising processes of advanced medical technologies and global information systems. Within this formulation of the body death becomes less central, bodies are spatialised, colonised and commodified. Nurses, like other therapeutic agents, can engage in educational and therapeutic roles aimed at enhancing people's self surveillance. The body as living flesh, by contrast, is a metaphor aimed at capturing the atextual body as it may be experienced through embodied communication in the context of understandings about embodied frailty and vulnerability.

In postmodernity, nursing itself is being constituted as text within the rapidly changing 'post institutional' structures of health care as it shifts away from the hierarchies and medical dominance of modernity into the competing contested terrains of postmodernity. Nursing becomes one set of information in processes dominated increasingly by economic rationalism. Nevertheless, within these structures spaces are opened up between competing discourses of postmodernity. Here nurses may be uneasily positioned in the present at the edge of beyond, in a disoriented and disturbed space. However, these spaces also allow for critical distance from dominant discourses; for reflection, humility, cautious action and the possibility of the emergence of new understandings.

REFERENCES

Benhabib S 1990 Epistemologies of postmodernism: a rejoinder to Jean-Francois Lyotard. In: Nicholson L J (ed) Feminism/postmodernism. Routledge, New York

Bergson H 1965 Duration and simultaneity. Bobbs Merrill, New York

Bhabha H K 1994 The location of culture. Routledge, London

Butler J 1993 Bodies that matter: on the discursive limits of 'sex'. Routledge, New York

Foucault M 1980 Michel Foucault: power/knowledge: selected interviews and other writings, 1972–1977. Harvester press, Brighton

Grosz E 1994 Volatile bodies: toward a corporeal feminism. Allen & Unwin, St Leonards

Habermas J 1983 Modernity — an incomplete project. In: Foster H (ed) Postmodern culture, Pluto Press, London

Haraway D 1990 A manifesto for cyborgs: science, technology and socialist feminism in the 1980s. In: Nicholson L J (ed) Feminism/post modernism. Routledge, New York

Hartsock N 1990 Foucault on power: a theory for women? In: Nicholson L J (ed) Feminism/postmodernism. Routledge, New York, 157–175

Heller A, Feher F 1988 The postmodern political condition. Polity Press, Cambridge

Illich I 1986 Body history (unpublished paper)

Ingham A 1989 A review of the literature relating to touch and its use in intensive care. Intensive Care Nursing 5:65–75

Lawler J 1991 Behind the screens: nursing, somology and the problem of the body. Churchill Livingstone, Melbourne

Leder D (ed) 1992 A tale of two bodies: the cartesian corpse and the lived body. In: The body in medical thought and practice. Kluwer Academic Publishers, Netherlands, 17–35

Levin D M, Solomon G F 1990 The discursive formation of the body in the history of medicine. Journal of Medicine and Philosophy 15:515–537

Lyotard J F 1984 The postmodern condition: a report on knowledge. Translated by G Bennington and B Massumi. University of Minneapolis Press, Minneapolis

Merleau-Ponty M 1962 The phenomenology of perception. Translated by C Smith. Routledge & Kegan Paul, London

Merleau-Ponty M 1968 The visible and the invisible. Northwestern University Press, Evanston

Owens C. 1993 The discourse of others: feminists and postmodernism. In: Foster H (ed) Postmodern culture. Pluto Press, London

Park Y 1983 Merleau-Ponty's ontology of the wild being. In: Tymieniecka A T (ed) Analecta Husserliana 16:313–326

Parker J M, Gardner G 1992 The silence and silencing of the nurses' voice: a reading of patient progress notes. Australian Journal of Advanced Nursing 9(2):3–9

Price M J 1993 Exploration of body listening: health and physical self awareness in chronic illness. Advances In Nursing Science 15(4):37–52

Quinn J F, Strelkauskas A J 1993 Psychoimmunlogic effects of therapeutic touch on practitioners and recently bereaved recipients: a pilot study. Advances in Nursing Science 15(4):13–26

Trinh T Minh-Ha 1992 Framer framed, Routledge, New York

Wilkes E 1994 Introduction. In: Clark D (ed) The future of palliative care: issues in policy and practice. Open University Press, Buckingham

Wiltshire J, Parker J M 1996 Containing abjection in nursing: the end of shift handover as a site of containment. Nursing Inquiry 3(1):23–29

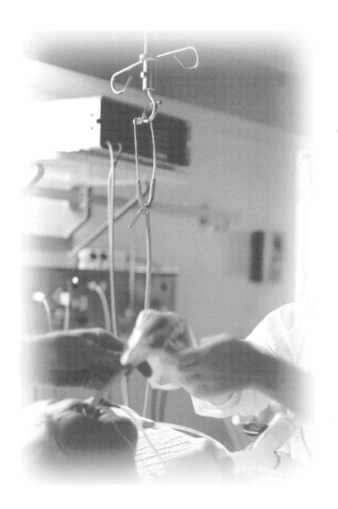

4

Knowing the body and embodiment
Methodologies, discourses and nursing

Jocalyn Lawler

Introduction

In this chapter I would like to consider the issue of how we, as relative newcomers to the formal academy, are being invited to formalise our knowing and researching of the body and embodiment within dominant discourses. It is my argument that our knowing and our discourse(s) should both reflect and affect the manner of our practice as nurses. However, our recorded discourses and formalised knowing are more reflective of influences external to nursing than the practice of nursing as it might emerge from clinical practice settings.

The central question I want to explore here is this: how are we, as nurses, to know and understand the body and embodiment as researchable topics of fundamental importance to the discipline? I am taking it as self-evident that the body and embodiment *are* central concerns of nursing.

The physical body is studied, in pieces, in a number of different disciplines, but embodiment has attracted much less attention. Where embodiment (the experience of the lived body) has been studied, it has been predominantly a topic for philosophy inquiry in which matters of the intellect and consciousness have been central. Embodiment in its more encompassing sense (beyond the intellect) has a history as a relatively silent and ignored matter, unlike the object body. There are two main reasons why this has been the case: first, dominant discourses of the modern period have submerged the subjective in the quest for objective and 'value free' (pure) knowledge; and second, the academy, which is powerfully masculinsed, has found topics such as emotions and feelings to be troublesome (Lawler 1991a).

As we have moved more into the realm of the postmodern, which focuses (in part) on the human subject(ive), scholars in feminism, sociology, and nursing are looking more comprehensively at the embodied realm of human existence. They are looking beyond consciousness, thinking and rational thought, to explore hitherto marginalised and moralised domains (see for example *Sexy Bodies*, Grosz & Probyn 1996, which emphasises the carnal experiences of feminism).

Nursing knowledge and much of its practice have been silenced and rendered relatively invisible because of 'the problem of the body' and this is a function of two things: first, knowledges of the body have been theoretically and epistemologically fragmented; and second, our cultures and way of life have rendered the body private and unspeakable (Lawler 1990, 1991b:1-3). I want to re-visit and extend my earlier discussion of the problem of the body by focusing on the discourses and disciplinary practices that help sustain epistemological fragmentation, in particular the positivist discourses of science and economics. It will be my argument that, as discourses which take the stance of objectivity, they necessarily submerge the personal and subject(ive); and that, as disciplines which hinge on what is quantifiable, they make it difficult for us to formalise our knowing about embodiment and nursing. That aspect of the problem of the body, which relates to the private and taboo nature of nursing work, will not be discussed in any detail here.

My discussion draws on Foucault's notions of power/knowledge and 'games of truth' as they are embedded in, and mediated by, typifying practices within and among the formal disciplines in the academy. Games of truth were described by Foucault as 'an ensemble of rules for the production of the truth'; the resultant 'truth' itself is, therefore, a function of the rules and principles of its production and inseparable from the discourses employed to communicate it (see Foucault's interview with Fornet-Betancourt et al in *The Final Foucault* 1988).

The tensions which surround the question of how to articulate nursing's knowledges[1] of the body and embodiment (and other aspects of our discipline) centre on which games of truth will best render nursing known, knowable, and researchable. We have three identifiable means from which to chose and through which we have operated with varying degrees of success: (i) the biomedical sciences and scientific discourses generally, including the social sciences, which are all predominantly derived from the academy and sustained by it; (ii) economically driven discourses that pervade the market place and the state; and (iii) practising nursing and reflecting on it. The first two of these are positivistic, reductive, predictive and probabilistic; in that they are alike and indistinguishable. However, knowing derived from practising nursing and reflecting on it and from studies of the experience of illness and embodiment are emerging as narrative in form, irreducible, personalised, contextual, and meaningful only as a gestalt; these ways of knowing are not necessarily predictive or probabilistic.

While the discourses and disciplinary practices of the biomedical and social sciences offer nursing ways to articulate its knowledges, which are relatively useful and helpful, they are not entirely adequate. What economics offers nursing as a practice based discipline is less appealing and potentially damaging. What I want to focus on here is the tension between, and choices inherent in, articulating (or performing) our knowing in these different and differing ways.

Scientific discourses, the problem of the body, and knowing in nursing

The 'traditional' sciences, which have their origins in the academy, pursue knowledge, often for its own sake; in this sense, the sciences and nursing are in sympathy with each other in so far as nursing seeks to validate itself by articulating a discrete body of knowledge. On other matters, predominantly methodologies and models of knowing, nursing and the sciences have less in common. Nursing knowledges, like many other knowledges, can be made to look familiar to those who are accustomed to positivist/scientific discourses. And we might also, perhaps, use their terminology and conceptual bases; in many respects, we already do, particularly in areas where we share common concerns, for example, in areas such as anatomy, physiology, biochemistry and the workings of the material world. But turning nursing into look-alike scientific knowledge can be misleading and it can construct epistemic falsehoods that are to nursing's disadvantage.

Most particularly, we want to know about what takes place between the nurse and the patient as people who are often situated as captives together. The patient is captive in the dysfunctional and/or sick(ly) body or with an embodied problem[2] and the nurse is captive with the patient, often for hours or days on end, or until death occurs. As captives, their worlds are necessarily brought together and focused on more immediate concerns and on ways in which experiences can be endured and transcended. It is possible to understand some of these experiences, both for the patient and the nurse, within the conceptual and discursive space of captivity about which we know little except in so far as it relates to matters over which the state presides.

The practice of nursing relies on many different ways of knowing and many kinds of knowledge nursing knowledges. Consequently, the nature of nursing knowledges and emerging disciplinary practices mean that borrowings, while necessary, will not suffice for nursing because so much of what we know comes from both being a nurse and doing nursing; that is, nursing's knowledges are ontological (and felt), intellectual, performed and expressed. Therefore, we want and need to talk differently about some of the same things that concern disciplines with which we share those common concerns and whose methodologies and discourses we have borrowed and, at times, appropriated.

Knowing, scientific discourses, the body and embodiment

I would like to make some observations about the multiple meanings of the verb, to know, and its adjectival form, knowing, that we might consider in the light of how we want to know the body and embodiment in nursing. The verb, *to know*, is said to mean:

> 1. to perceive or understand as fact or truth, or apprehend with clearness and certainty ... [or] 2. to have fixed in the mind or memory; *to know a poem by heart* ... [or] 3. to be cognisant or aware of; to be acquainted with (a thing, place, person etc.), as by sight, experience, or report ... [or] 4. to understand from experience or attainment [e.g.] ... how to make something ... [or] 5. to be able to distinguish, as one from another ... [or] 6. **not to know from Adam,** not to recognise (someone) ... [or] 7. **know chalk from cheese,** to be able to note differences ... [or] 8. **know the ropes** ... to know the details or methods of any business or the like etc. (*The Macquarie Dictionary* 1991).

There are several observations that can be highlighted in these forms of knowing. First, the research community does not equally value these different forms; second, some ways to know are sensitive to context, experience(s) and the passage of time; third, some are inherently unstable and changeable[3] while others are more enduring and robust;[4] and fourth, some forms can be expressed in language and others cannot. However, those forms which can be encased in language are the most pervasive and, according to Foucault, the most powerful. Also, some forms of knowledge are affected by our memories, cognitive/intellectual activities (or decline), readings and research, and others change only in relation to life circumstances, periods of emotional turbulence, profound shocks, and examination of self and the meaning of life. Yet we live in a world that places relatively more value on forms of knowledge which can be externalised, verbalised, and often in nursing — proselytised, if not evangelised! As economic rationalism and late-stage capitalism manifest themselves in the so-called 'information' age, knowledge has also become a commodity to be commercialised and traded.

The adjectival form *knowing* takes on more subtle and socially constructed qualities than the verb *to know*, but again with a relatively dominant emphasis on the intellect. For example, *knowing* is said to mean:

> 1. shrewd, sharp, or astute; often affecting or suggesting shrewd or secret understanding of matters: *a knowing glance.* 2. having knowledge or information; intelligent; wise. 3. conscious; intentional; deliberate (*The Macquarie Dictionary* 1991).

We cannot talk of knowing and knowledge in isolation from *what* we know; nor can we ignore the social significance and political consequences of that knowing. I want to turn now to that issue and focus on the several questions: (i) what do we know about the body and embodiment?; (ii) how have we come to know them and render them knowable matters; (iii) how do we talk about them?; (iv) what do we know that we do not or cannot admit to our formal discourses; and (v) what have we silenced?

If knowledge is both the source of power and inseparable from it and the discourses which mediate it (Foucault 1980), our knowledges of the body and embodiment are indeed powerful. However, our knowing has been, and continues to be, affected by regulation and control often through its transformation into dominant discourses which are recognised and respected in the academy but which are not necessarily inherently suited to nursing. In another context, I have argued that

> Academic traditions of western patriarchy create illusions about knowledge and ways to know which make nursing seem inherently untidy. Nursing is concerned with things, like feelings and emotions and the body, which the academy has difficulty accommodating ... [A]spects of the human condition which make people uncomfortable, but which are central concerns of nursing, are in danger of being marginalised and disenfranchised because the traditions of the academy operate to transform them into something less threatening to the established order.
>
> As a consequence of the dominant ideas of that established order in the academy, nursing has been presented with a kind of 'Sophie's choice' about the location of its knowledge and the methods which may be used to articulate and research that knowledge. Nurses have been asked to choose between the seeable and the feelable ... [but we] must address both lived and material reality (Lawler 1991a:13).

We have many more opportunities to formalise our knowing and teaching (see Brown & Seddon 1996) of the physical body as a biological and medical entity than we do as embodiment or the-person-in-the-body because the latter are inherently subjective. Typically, scientific discourse relies heavily on a form of objectivity which invites distance and detachment rather than engagement with the subjective — in effect excluding or minimising the potential effect(s) of the subjective. In this kind of knowing space, the body is the object of examination, inspection, and investigation as a physical thing like any other mechanical and biophysical machine whose malfunctions are identified and corrected. Running repairs and replacements are the order of things — much like a motor vehicle — as long as you can get the replacement parts or fix the original ones, you can keep the machine going. If we, as nurses, want and need to know the human body in this way, and we do in some respects, how are we to relate our knowledge of it to others and what will be the manner of our discourse?

If nursing evolves its disciplinary practices and discourses for knowing of the body in terms which typify the natural and biomedical sciences, the body will be anonymous, de-personalised, passive, and, inevitably, reduced to the sum of its malfunctioning parts and related remedies. Furthermore, embodiment will not feature at all. Those are the inescapable consequences because the methodologies and discourses of these sciences would invite us and, seemingly, demand of us that we research and record our knowledge of the physical body in this way (see Parker & Gardner 1992).

To illustrate my point, I will turn to a report on events which are, in some respects, medical mistakes but which are reported, in Australia, as adverse drug reactions (Adverse Drug Reactions Advisory Committee 1994:2–3). I am referring to the gel, Dinoprostone (Prostin E2 Vaginal Gel) which was recently approved '...for induction of labour in pregnant women at or near term who have favourable induction features and who have a singleton pregnancy with a vertex presentation' (p.2). The report continues:

To October 1993...[the Committee] had received 5 reports of suspected uterine reactions associated with dinoprostone. Four of these reports described uterine perforation, which in 2 women, led to hysterectomy. In at least 2 of these cases, dinoprostone was not used in accordance with the approved indications.

In one case uterine rupture occurred about 2 hours after application of the gel whereas in another case it occurred more than 24 hours later. In a third case, although no uterine hypertonia was detected clinically, fetal bradycardia and persistent transverse lie (contraindicated) necessitated laparotomy. It was then found that uterine rupture had occurred intrapartum and the baby was lying within the mother's abdomen. In the fourth case, dinoprostone was administered twice to a woman who had a previous delivery by Caesarean section (contraindicated). Abdominal pain and fetal bradycardia led to an emergency Caesarean section with delivery of a stillborn baby and the observation that the uterine scar had ruptured. In a further report, although there was no uterine rupture, the patient experienced 4 hours of myometrial hypercontractility and hypertonus after the application of the gel (Adverse Drug Reactions Advisory Committee 1994:2).

There are many aspects of this report which invite critique and comment. However, I want to highlight the way in which these events are related to us — the readers and potential knowers about 'adverse drug reactions'. First, and most obviously, this is a relatively typical report of scientific/medical findings, albeit in the context of 'adverse drug reactions'. Second, the discourse is typically scientific; it is objective, precise, descriptive, and informative. Third, the narrative appears in third person passive prose — we know only that this is a story of 'adverse' events involving women in an advanced state of pregnancy. We do not know anything else about them; they have no personas and no distinguishing features except for the particular bodily arrangements of two of the women which constitute contraindications. These are not women in the more complete sense of the word; rather, they are cases of women's pregnant bodies and the bodies of babies, one of which is dead.

The manner of the reporting speaks to the scientific community and in that sense, it is unremarkable. Another reading of this report of 'adverse drug reactions' raises this question: in what way does the discourse of this report differentiate these women from cases involving any other large mammal — a sheep, a cow, a horse? If we want to know the body as a physical and physiological entity, are we, as nurses, also obliged to articulate our knowledge impersonally, objectively, dispassionately, and with detachment? What are the consequences if we do, and what are the consequences if we do not? Is there a space between these two epistemological and discursive worlds?

It is reasonable to assume that the experience of myometrial hyper-contractility and hypertonus is both painful and distressing, but the manner of the reporting does not allow for the ontological features of these conditions to be discussed because the subjective is silenced. We read nothing of the pain, distress and suffering of these women because the reported events are contextualised not around the women, but the drug. If there is such little space for the subject(ive) in the scientised knowledge/discourse of biomedicine, what, if any space does it allow for the subject(ive) in practice?

The most remarkable aspect of this report, however, is that the gel is constituted as the causal agent, and not the person or persons who prescribed it. And it is safe to assume, in these cases, that self-medication is not an issue. If we read this report with a view to the properties of narrative (see Polkinghorne 1988) we are invited by the manner of the discourse in the report to ascribe agentivity to the gel, leaving silent the matter of who prescribed and/or administered it.

However, if we take Kenneth Burke's view, we would read this story differently; he argued that 'well-formed stories ... are composed of a pentad of an actor [or actors], an action, a goal, a scene, and an instrument — plus trouble' (Kenneth Burke 1945 cited in Bruner 1990:50). So, if we read about these 'adverse drug reactions' from the perspective of Burke's description of a good story, we would re-cast the gel not as the agent, but as the instrument. Who then, we might ask, is the actor? If we view the discourse of this report from a narrative frame of reference, we render the objectivity of scientific discourse problematic for disciplines such as nursing, which are concerned with human experience, embodiment and intersubjective interaction.

It is not my argument that biomedicine is inherently unconcerned with the human condition; rather, it is to propose that the manner of a typifying and dominant discourse is reflective of typifying and dominant practice. In the case of medical practice, allegiance to the rational-scientific model, with its emphasis on practising on the physical, object(ive) world, has led to dehumanising trends when applied to the object(ive) body of the patient — a pattern of medical care that some of their own profession have criticised (see, for example, Kleinman 1988, Moore 1991, Little 1995). Kleinman has argued, for example, that '... a medical or scientific perspective ... doesn't help us to deal with the problem of suffering' (1988:28). It would be possible to re-read Kleinman's statement to mean that these perspectives do not deal with embodiment; nor does the discourse of biomedicine allow for it as a mainstream concern. The same can be said of the discourse of economics in so far as it is being used to structure misleading language and thinking about nursing practice(s), which I will address later in this chapter.

Scientific reporting, the person(al), and third person passive prose

Scientific discourse does not allow the person to enter the story, except in the passive voice and, consequently, it does not allow for embodiment or the non-material world. In that sense, therefore, scientific methodologies, in so far as they are inseparable from the discourses which typify them, are inadequate for nursing; they may allow us to know the body, but not in a way which provides space for an understanding of embodiment — and I argue that we cannot have one without the other (Lawler 1991b). Scientific discourse is inadequate for nursing's understanding of the body as a physical thing because we do not have the ideological, practical, philosophical or epistemological liberty to stand apart and distant from it; nursing is also concerned with the embodied other as a human being and that concern is interactive, contextual and intersubjective.

Put another way, if nursing is a form of practice in which the object and experienced body are integrated in the context of particular patients and their nursing care (Lawler 1991b), such matters cannot adequately be conveyed in the discourse typical of scientific reporting. Not only does a scientific perspective, unlike nursing, place primary emphasis on the physical body and the physical (non-experiential) world generally, it is conducted in third person passive prose; and this form of prose reflects the assumption that, in science, objectivity is a necessary condition for good research.

Another example from the literature highlights the same problem of scientific/medical methodologies and discourses as they apply in psychiatry, which is, presumably, a little closer to the person and a little more resistant to distancing discourse. The case report, which I use to illustrate this point concerns a young Ethiopian woman who became anorexic following a period of imprisonment and torture (Fahy et al 1988). The report tells us that she is 22 years old, 157 centimetres tall and that, at the time of admission, she weighed 39 kilograms. Her history included vomiting, which began at the age of 16 when she was imprisoned, interrogated and tortured about the involvement of her father and brother in political activities. She was imprisoned for six months, during which time her father was executed and she was subjected to beatings and 'on one occasion, a blood-stained rag was stuffed into her mouth to prevent her screaming' (p.385). After this event, she had 'vomited blood-streaked material and when she attempted to eat, vomited repeatedly. She said that at the time, eating had reminded her of the rag in her mouth' (p.385).

The report continues to detail her medical, psychiatric and life histories which included: weight loss, 'abnormal eating and vomiting'; work with refugees; qualifying as a pharmacist; and her migration to the UK where she came to the attention of the group who eventually reported her case in the literature. The report contains a brief section called 'investigations' in which we are told that 'on physical examination, extensive scarring was found across both her breasts. There were scars on her elbows and dorsal surfaces of the feet from previous lash-injuries'. She had a number of other investigations of her gastrointestinal system, a CAT scan of her head, and a psychometric assessment including an assessment of her attitudes to eating.[5] All were within normal limits. We are then told relatively more about her mental state and progress, that she was placed on an antidepressant medication, and that there was 'a nursing regime of a kind formulated for patients with anorexia nervosa, but in this case beginning with a liquid diet' (pp.385–6).

While not wanting to take this report out of context — because it is principally concerned with reporting an unusual and atypical aetiology for anorexia nervosa — the manner of the reporting is such that perforce, the woman's story is objectified and so is she. Allowing for the complexities of body/self interplays in anorexia nervosa and the authors' attention to details relevant to her social being, the reading which these authors — all men (in so far as one can tell from given names) — make of her condition and progress is taken predominantly from the physical body. We learn little about what meanings the woman makes of her experiences, diagnosis, situation or embodied being. The report reads as if the discourse of scientific/psychiatric reporting takes priority over the embodied experiences and subjective meanings which the woman herself might relate.

This is not a situation isolated to the scientific and medical communities, but one which is also apparent in the discourses which appear in some nursing literature. Such literature demonstrates the tensions between the customs of scientific and 'academic' reporting, which have been adopted to a greater or lesser extent in nursing, and matters in which the subject(ive) is central. This tension is most apparent in situations where third person passive prose is used to relate knowing in which the subjective experience of the other is the central theme. The mismatch between the chosen discourse for reporting and the subject matter it concerns often sounds quaint, if not superficial or artificial and possibly patronising. The central problem is quite simple: the phenomenon under investigation is subjective experience related to us in objective prose.

I have taken an example from *Nursing Science Quarterly* (Coward 1990) to demonstrate my point. This example illustrates the limitations of third person passive prose and the problems of 'objective' reporting for some ways of knowing in nursing. The report is titled, 'The lived experience of the self-transcendence in women with advanced breast cancer'. It was an exploratory study, the purpose of which was to describe women's experiences of self-transcendence, that is, reaching out beyond oneself. We are told in the article that:

> The research was planned and conducted using the phenomenological research method as described by Colaizzi (1978). The first step was for *the researcher* to examine *her* presuppositions about the topic to be investigated. In *her* experience with seriously ill patients, *she* had been puzzled by the considerable variation in the manner people faced illness [emphasis added] (Coward 1990:163).

We can ask: who is this anonymous person called 'the researcher'?; what is her intention — as a phenomenological researcher — in entering into the meaning world of the other?; is this how she wanted to tell this story or did she feel obliged, compelled or required to tell her story of this research from the detached viewpoint of the third person?; is this what she has been taught about the 'proper' way to represent herself as a researcher?; or was this the only way she could tell the story and get her work published?[6] These are not trivial questions; rather, they are fundamental issues about how we want to articulate and represent our practice and how we want to build our discourse and disciplinary practices in nursing.

When we, as nurses, use ourselves as the therapeutic agent in an interactive and person-to-person sense, scientific discourse is unavailable to us to articulate such matters publicly and formally; we — the practitioners — are relatively silent, silenced, and invisible. Third person passive prose creates distance, removes reference to the personal and subjective, and disallows the articulation of matters at the core of nursing practice. And that does not begin to address those aspects of nursing practice that cannot be framed in words, formalised, or encapsulated in *any* form of discourse because they are felt, perceived, experienced and known in an embodied and shared way.[7] However, while the discourses of biomedical and social sciences do not accommodate embodied and felt knowledge formally, they are recognised and acknowledged, albeit informally, peripherally, and inadequately. In economic discourse such recognition is usually absent.

Economic discourse, nursing, and the embodied other

I want to focus here on the impact on nursing of economically derived and economically driven discourses and disciplinary practices. Economic discourses, because they do not account for embodiment and personal meaning making, with which the experience of health and illness are centrally concerned, are inadequate[8] for, and detrimental to, the evolution of discourses for nursing practice. Also, as positivist approaches[9], they are methodologically inadequate for studying embodiment and nursing. Economic discourses and methodologies have distracted and misled us, and worse — have seduced us into formalising our knowing of the physical body and nursing care in a form which is more meaningful and useful to economists and managers than it is to practising nurses, scholars and researchers. Our knowledge of embodiment and our dealings with the person-in-the-body, however, cannot find an authentic and authenticable space in economic discourse and games of truth; that is another compelling reason to reject them as inadequate and inappropriate for nursing.

In the last three decades, the discourses, concerns and disciplinary practices of economics — especially economic rationalism — have gradually but progressively invaded our everyday social and working lives, language, daily news reports, media commentary and politicians' addresses on 'the state of the nation'. Some have argued that economic rationalism, in the western world in particular, has taken priority over political and social order — a trend unaccompanied by serious debate about its consequences (see Cordery 1995). Nursing and health care, like other public sector institutions, have been affected and, in some respects, transformed by economic rationalist philosophies, policies and practice(s) — also without much debate or sustained criticism.

In the contexts of the practice setting where the financial and resource management of clinical services is a major issue, nursing has virtually no viable alternative, in the current climate, than to adopt paradigms and discourses of market economics as the dominant means with which to articulate nursing matters when there is a need to communicate to non-nurses about resource issues. This is an economic imperative; without the means to speak about nursing in the language of economics, nursing is vulnerable to erosion and to relative impoverishment in the provision of nursing services.

Being able to communicate about nursing in economic discourse, however, does not guarantee protection from the erosion of nursing services both in numerical and other ways. In some respects it may contribute to erosion, especially if there is no acceptance of the extent to which aspects of nursing cannot be reduced to, or rendered meaningful as, entities that can be measured for productivity, cost effectiveness and efficiency. The question of value (and cost) in this context is operationalised in its monetary sense; the more generic and socially constructed notion of value is irrelevant in economic discourses, though it has a token presence in the rhetoric of 'quality care', 'best practice' and the like.

Problems of economic discourse and games of truth for nursing

At their most fundamental level, the purposes and intentions of economic games of truth and economically derived discourses are not the articulation of clinical matters so that we might better understand the practice of nursing. Rather, they are designed for cost control, the allocation of resources and the relatively arbitrary, but allegedly objective, business of assigning monetary values to factors which are constitutive of economic understandings of health care systems and their resource utilisation. Economically derived discourses, which pervade public discussion at the political level, also have been adopted and inculcated into the language and texts of nursing, most particularly those which originate in the USA. Such texts, however, are typically devoid of critiques which would problematise these trends and issues, and they show little sensitivity to the relevance of these writings in other countries or cultures (see Lawler 1991c). Rather, they tend to promote, 'sell', or more seriously, evangelise a particular viewpoint or way of thinking — and they are well placed to do that, given the extent to which works published in the USA saturate the international nursing literature.

It is one thing for us to borrow concepts, discourses and research methodologies to try out in nursing, or to respond pragmatically to a prevailing economic climate; it is another thing entirely to be subjected to the imposition of the discourses and methodologies of market economics on nursing which is, in many respects, concerned with matters that are embodied, interpersonal, socially constructed, human, and shared. Economically derived discourses, which underlie nursing process, nursing diagnoses, casemix, DRGs and much of the current thinking on quality in health care and outcome standards, are much more troublesome for nursing than are the biomedical and social sciences, for a number of reasons.

First, economic discourse invites us to adopt the language, concepts and methodologies of the market place to reflect matters which are clinical and practical; as a result, the practice of nursing is articulated within an imposed discourse which is not derived from the doing of nursing but from the perspective of measurement-for-the-sake-of-costing or outcome assessment. Nursing per se is not, therefore, articulated in a form inherently suited to it as a practice discipline, but in a discourse that reflects economic constructs and games of truth.

Second, within economic discourse and methodologies, nursing is at a particularly high risk because economics, like other disciplines which rely on positivist methodologies, leaves no space for many of the subtleties of nursing. Rather, important aspects of nursing practice, like aspects of the body and embodiment (see Lawler 1991b), are constituted by their absence and silence, or by a form of words that diminishes them. A good example of how nursing is diminished in this way can be found in Reeve's (1993) report, *Coherent & Consistent Quality Assurance & Utilisation Review Activities in Public and Private Hospitals in Australia*, in which he claims that:

> Casemix and Quality in nursing care will require careful overview of the costing process. Casemix will impact on the cost of nursing services. Sensitivity must be exercised as to the level at which this occurs. **It would not be difficult to eliminate the vital, personal elements of the art of nursing care. If costed too tightly, such a move could reduce the amount of time the nurse would have to just pass the time with a patient, a component of nursing that has been traditional and special to the profession. This would be a serious negative result for the Casemix programme which is designed to be a positive initiative. The matters need close attention. To overlook it would have serious consequences for the Quality of Care** (original emphasis) (Reeve 1993:46).

Reeve's report illustrates how we may not be able to speak of nursing in the language which is understood, or about things which are valued, by those who currently set the economic and political agenda (see Lawler 1993). What Reeve calls '... just pass[ing] time with a patient' is understood and articulated differently by nurses. Taylor's (1990, 1994) work on ordinariness and the interpersonal qualities in nursing and Marck's (1990) work on therapeutic reciprocity are two particularly relevant examples of how we, as nurses, understand 'pass[ing] the time' as interactive, contextual, richly grounded in knowing the other and intended for therapeutic effect. Nurses make known their knowledge of these subtle and sophisticated matters using words and language which do not diminish either the acts or actors themselves as they are related to us.

The third reason why economic discourse is troublesome for nursing is that the main agenda for economics is the aggregation of data which leaves little space for the individual and individual experience. This is a sad irony for nursing, given the extent of our investment in promoting individualised care as a central tenet of nursing and about which so much has been written and spoken. Much of the discourse about 'individualised' care, however, has been filtered through nursing process rhetoric which is, in itself, an inherently positivistic and economically driven construct and which does not allow for embodiment or lived experience more generally (Lawler 1991b, 1991c).

Fourth, economic discourses and practices do not benefit from the humbling and sobering realities that people in clinical practice understand. Economists' knowing, like that of the general scientific community, is a rather more impersonal affair, at least in so far as it is committed to the published record.

Effects of economic discourse on nursing practice

The methodologies which stem from economics, and economic rationalist philosophies in particular, emphasise efficiency and cost effectiveness in so far as they can be made meaningful as functions of positivist, cause-and-effect, outcome oriented models. Consequently, what counts as data are de-contextualised indicators by which efficiency and effectiveness can be assessed within the games of truth that typify economics. Cordery (1995) has been very critical of this approach, arguing that within economic rationalist methodologies

> [t]he rich and non reducible aspects of organised socioeconomic life — the things from which one develops a sense of identity and meaningful existence — are marginalised. This is a great irony for economic philosophy and theory, particularly when one considers the extent to which the social sciences generally — economics excepted — have moved into the postmodernist era and recognised the limitations of positivist understandings of social order (p.357)

In Foucault's terms (1988), the games of truth within economic rationalist methodology are self-contained, circular, and apparently self-serving — and they are distinctly and powerfully modern at a time when other disciplines move to postmodern ways of knowing. In the language and methodologies of the economists and accountants, the non-quantifiable aspects of nursing, or those qualities of practice which cannot readily be measured and factored into output-oriented formulae, are particularly vulnerable. In part, this is due to what van Manen (1990:113) called *epistemological silence*, that is, 'the kind of silence we are confronted with when we face the unspeakable'.

Epistemological silence has several forms, but the form of interest to nursing, in relation to the games of truth within economics, concerns the manner in which some things are sensitive to the discourse in which they are related. This sensitivity can be illustrated by using the concept of love, which is problematic for behavioural science methodologies and discourse, but not for the discursive forms used in poetry, music and the fine arts (van Manen 1990:114–115). The same could be said of the different discursive forms employed to describe what nurses do when they talk with patients. In the economic discourse which Reeve (1993) uses, nurses' talk with patients is constituted as 'just pass[ing] the time with the patient'; but grounded in a nursing discourse, such talk becomes the rich and valuable concepts of therapeutic reciprocity (Marck 1990), ordinariness (Taylor 1990, 1994), making ordinary (Parker & Gardner 1992) and creating an environment of permission (Lawler 1991b), among other things which are yet to be articulated. Not surprisingly, these works by nurses were all conducted within interpretive paradigms and discourses and their data are in narrative form.

What nurses talk with patients about includes a wide range of apparently normal, and highly 'abnormal' subject matter which, in its own right, is worthy of serious investigation (see, for example Bottorff & Varcoe 1995). However, the interactive and interpersonal qualities of talk(ing) itself help to transform extraordinary situations in which patients are vulnerable, uncertain, and fearful, into states which can be endured, transcended, survived, or from which it is possible to recover; such states usually centre around the dysfunctions and disfigurements of the physical body and distresses of human embodiment, fear of death, disease or the person's ability to endure suffering. These are not topics about which one 'just pass[es] the time of day' as though it is small talk of no great consequence beyond sociability.

The discourse and methodologies of economics have had a dramatic, but under-recognised, impact on nursing. Coming as they did after a period of sustained pressure to scientise nursing knowledge, economically driven constructs of nursing which are themselves based on the fundamentals of scientific methodology are just another indication of attempts to authenticate nursing within a basically patriarchal world. I have criticised this trend previously, arguing that

> [t]he academic discourse on the discipline [of nursing], which is dominated by the USA, has reflected a growing emphasis on the perceived 'need' to develop and scientise nursing knowledge. We have been encouraged — extolled even — by most of the North Americans and their Australian followers to embrace positivist scientific models, and with them reduction, objectification, quantification and taxonomic and linear thinking. We have been encouraged to see scientific knowledge and scientific nursing practices as universal and highly desirable features of the discipline — indeed some have gone so far as to argue that it is only through traditionally scientific methods that we can develop the knowledge base and standing (that is, the status) of the discipline. While much of nursing practice can be studied by quantification, measurement and positivist inquiry, individual patient perspectives and perceptions are also important, especially if we are committed to patient-centred care. But within positivist approaches patients' experiences of illness can become peripheral or unresearchable. Although nursing has, of necessity, accommodated more technologically and scientifically oriented health care, it has also retained a concern for the care and comfort of patients but, in the academic literature, this commitment has taken on some ideological, rhetorical and philosophical qualities as notions of 'scientific' nursing have tended to override non-quantifiable elements in nursing (Lawler 1991c:214).

Dunlop's (1986) critique of how the quest to scientise the concept of caring is a classic example of how science — for the sake of science itself — has contributed to thinking and lines of argument that cannot be sustained in nursing; they are nonsensical and philosophically and epistemologically incoherent. Furthermore, attempting to scientise nursing, ipso facto, risks a potentially damaging transformation of concerns central to nursing. In the short term, and perhaps more importantly, scientising nursing can create the impression — however erroneously and unintended — either that there is little of substance in nursing practice or that nursing is another scientific approach to health care. Not all of nursing or human responses to, or experiences of, illness and health care can be explained with reference to positivist models of knowing nor within scientific or economic discourse; rather, we also look to storytelling, narrative knowing, aesthetics and personal meaning making as ways in which our worlds and practice can speak to us and for us.

The 'new' nursing language, embodiment and the body

Economically motivated demands to demonstrate nursing's effect on patient care are apparent not only in more global constructs such as the nursing process and nursing diagnosis but also in the language that accompanies them. This language is not an authentic nursing discourse but an economically derived dialect that reflects the influence of economic games of truth on nursing.

The term, 'high dependency nursing', for example, is one of the earliest terms which is inherently economic; it derives originally from measurement of the level of nursing time required for particular categories of patients whose physical body — and what needs to be done to it by nurses — are the sources from which temporally defined demands originate. The term does not speak to particular nursing practices nor a substantive area of our knowledge base, necessarily, but to the notion of quantifiable time as it can be measured in minutes. In practice, however, high dependency nursing has come to mean a number of things to nurses and we have developed some shared sense of what a high dependency unit or patient is; the problem is that we have not yet found a more epistemologically or ontologically authentic term to replace it and, in doing so, liberate us from the language of time-and-money.

However, nursing diagnoses provide the best example not only of the imposition of economic discourse and language on nursing but also the false assumptions about the utility, for nursing, of inclusive, logico-linear and output-oriented models. Without entering into the debates about their questionable ethicality (Mitchell 1991), cultural insensitivity and North American bias (Lawler 1991c), lack of clinical support (Dennison & Keeling 1989), and restrictive, narrow focus (Mitchell & Santopinto 1988), there are questions about their validity and conceptual clarity (Jenny 1987). More importantly, there are questions about what they exclude and silence, and whom they oppress. One particularly curious example of this pressure to 'diagnose' patients' nursing needs is the (unofficial) nursing diagnosis of 'acopia'[10] that has evolved in at least one Australian hospital. This 'condition' is manifested in a variety of ways, all of which are indicative of normal human responses to suffering and distress but which cannot be addressed within the (economically determined) resources of the nursing staff. In the context of nursing diagnoses, normality is pathologised and rendered 'a problem', in a way reminiscent of psychology's attempts to deal with coping behaviour (see Wortmann & Silver 1989). An 'acopic' patient (or relative) is often one who requires emotional support or whose lived body experience is the source of most angst.

Advocates of nursing diagnosis themselves admit that 'the implementation of nursing diagnosis in the clinical area continues to produce resistance, duplication and frustration ... [but that] since the early 1980s, [it has] been used with increasing frequency and consistency in periodicals, textbooks, and nursing care plans' (Vincent & Coler 1990). There is, as yet, no evidence that the advent of nursing diagnosis is improving care, facilitating the work of clinicians or in any way enhancing the articulation of nursing knowledge. Rather, we are witnessing a re-run of the pattern that typified the introduction of the nursing process, which has itself been a spectacular failure when assessed against its own alleged benefits. Not only are these economically generated notions alien to practitioners, but they are also imposed, usually by the same people who write the texts and promote the use of care plans to which Vincent and Coler (1990) refer. In terms of the more global picture, the imposition of nursing diagnosis configures the research-practice nexus 'arsy-versy' (Lawler 1991c). As a consequence, nursing, as it might emerge from clinical practice, is silenced and marginalised, and issues of central importance to patients, such as how they might interpret what is happening to them, are not afforded a space.

One of the major areas of silence is embodiment — and there are some clear and quite straightforward explanations for that. The most obvious reason is that the concept of nursing diagnosis is derived from within a biomedical and traditional scientific-reductive paradigm where the focus is the physical world, including the physical body, and on what can be observed and measured; it is also a model of rational knowledge, which necessarily excludes non-cognitive-intellectual ways of knowing. There is no real problem here, for nursing, in so far as the physical body and its biophysical malfunctions and remedies are concerned, because nursing is inescapably concerned, among other things, with the physical body and its malfunctions.

However, the biophysical model does not and cannot claim to account for aspects of practice which are contextually dependent or which have their origins within the person-in-the-body and his or her embodied experiences of illness, disease and health care. These are limitations that are not acknowledged by advocates of nursing diagnostics or health economists as important indicators of care or quality of nursing.

The real danger of nursing diagnosis lies in the false premise that it is an inclusive and comprehensive taxonomy, which potentially can account for nursing; such a proposition is untenable and excessive. For example, in their argument to introduce a unified diagnostic model for nursing, Vincent and Coler (1990) construct their case for integrating NANDA and ANA taxonomies, in part, with very selective reference to what happens in biology. What they fail to take into account is that taxonomies in biology are based on anatomy and anatomical differences, that is, physical difference. Unlike nursing, biological taxonomies do not attempt to include experiential or socially mediated phenomena. On that basis also, nursing diagnoses are manifestly inadequate as a comprehensive and inclusive taxonomic system.

Not surprisingly, the most controversial and problematic areas for developers of nursing diagnoses are those beyond biomedical parameters and the physical body, that is, the area of human responses to illness. There is a voluminous and compelling literature on the limitations of traditional scientific models for understanding humans and social life — literature that seems to have been ignored by those who continue to concoct and promote nursing diagnostics, interventions, and therapeutics.

46

More alarming, perhaps, is the use of the language of nursing diagnostics system as metaphors for nursing itself. The term 'nursing interventions', for example, is rapidly becoming a metaphor for nursing care, and consequently, nursing is in danger of being reduced (in terms both of its valuableness and in relation to methodology) to the sum of its repertoire of 'interventions'. There are several issues to be considered in this context: first, not all nursing can be captured in terms of interventions; and second, sometimes the best 'intervention' is not to intervene. On a more general level, speaking of nursing in the language of intervention is to suggest that nursing is inherently about intervening; whereas nursing is also about watching, waiting, and allowing nature to take its course. Nursing is about working with naturally occurring processes and is fundamentally a form of non-invasive practice. The term, 'interventions' is not a naturally derived notion in relation to nursing. Stripped of the things that nurses do at the behest of medicine or because of medical intervention, there is very little about nursing that is either invasive or interventionist.

Like other manifestations of economic rationalism in action, the games of truth of nursing diagnosis are self-contained, circular, and apparently self-serving. More importantly, they disempower and silence people on whom the games of truth are visited; this is reflected in Mitchell's (1991) argument that 'the diagnostic process encourages a professional arrogance which for some nurses is oppressive, restrictive and discomforting'. However, if one takes on nursing diagnostics, it is a 'package deal' along with managed care and other economically derived concepts about efficiency and effectiveness, which seemingly leaves nothing to chance. The package consists of the diagnosis itself to which interventions are assigned and measured as 'outcomes' — and all this is situated in the context of what is believed to be the province of care in which nursing is the accountable profession.

Nursing, however, is an inherently untidy discipline which has to straddle a very wide range of paradigms, knowledges, problems and daily contingencies and demands (Lawler 1991c); it is not, therefore, amenable to inclusive models in which everything is neat and tidy. There is another problem which is rather difficult to pin down, and that is a direct result of the games of truth which nursing diagnosis employs. The problem created by the game goes like this: if the phenomena of concern to nursing are those things which can be framed in nursing diagnoses, and if the nurse is accountable only for those things which lie within the phenomena of concern to nursing, then where does that leave those aspects of nursing practice which cannot be reflected in this non-inclusive, but allegedly inclusive, model.

How does nursing address those things which do not lend themselves to logico-linear, positivistic, rational, outcome-oriented, causal models; where does that leave meaning making, storytelling, embodiment and the embodied self — and where does that leave the patients' perspective? Taking the rhetoric and discourse of nursing diagnostics at face value, such matters must, by default, lie outside the domain of nursing as they define it. Such a proposition is a nonsense and it is dangerous.

Silencing discourses, games of truth and the emergence of nursing's voice

There are aspects of the ambience and environment in which nursing takes place, which can profoundly affect patient care, but which cannot be factored into outcome-driven economic formulae; nor can they be framed in economic or scientific discourses; nor can they be disaggregated to display patient care cost at the level of the individual. There is research evidence (for example, Shields 1978, Lawler 1994) that patients take great comfort from the perceived availability of the nurse. Availability is a perceived and intangible phenomenon that relates not only to the physical availability of the nurse, but also an emotional, personal, existential availability in which patients sense that the nurse is there for them — as the embodied and vulnerable 'other' who needs protection, reassurance and support. These are things that lie outside the discourse and modalities through which economic understandings are formalised.

Likewise, availability is not a concept which can be reflected in, or talked about, as an 'intervention' in the discourse of nursing diagnostics; nor would a hypothetical nursing diagnosis 'potential to need the availability of the nurse' have much credibility because such availability is implicit in the generic provision of a nursing service. Perceiving the availability of the nurse is an embodied and interpreted sense of safety and comfort that the patient experiences; it is not necessarily a rational event but an emotional response to felt states such as fear and vulnerability. Availability, in its felt sense, does not and cannot feature in economic or scientific models of nursing.

Evidence is also emerging that the dominant discursive form about clinical nursing matters, e.g. for verbal reports, is predominantly storytelling (Parker, Gardner & Wiltshire 1992). Furthermore, there are games of truth in reporting nursing which not only silence nursing but preserve the power of medicine to pronounce various biophysical events; that nurses also know how to pronounce is taken for granted, but silenced (Parker & Gardner 1992).

When we reflect on how are we to read and research nursing and draw some preliminary conclusions about how to read the physical body, lived body, the embodied self, experiences of illness and embodiment in nursing, we are left with some clear options. At the very least, we have a need to understand biophysical and biological events that affect the physical body and to do so in their discourses of origin — without that form of knowing and communication we would lose our points of anchorage with other aspects of health care. Because we also practise with living, breathing, speaking, social humans, we have a need to operate with reference to the humanities and the social sciences and to be able to speak their languages, without which we lose our points of anchorage to forms of knowing that focus on being human and embodied. Because we are schooled within western traditions, we have a need to face our ignorance of other ways of knowing and experiencing life, death, suffering and healing.

And because we are fundamentally a practice discipline and have a need to speak within, from and to the practice of nursing, we have a need to give voice to our own business. In that sense, much of nurses' business is a like women's business — it is taken for granted, it is storied, it is grounded in experiential knowing, and it has been silenced in a patriarchal world. We cannot render the body and embodiment researchable for nursing within borrowed methodologies, but we can — and have a need to — share in those knowledges in order to practise. We also have a need to see the limitations of what we borrow, or have imposed on us, and to explore ways of knowing — and ways to transmit that knowing to others — so that we reflect nursing and not nursing-through-the-words-of-others.

It is my argument that the discourses of the sciences and economics, while they have shaped and continue to shape the way we talk and think about nursing, have silenced important and central concerns for nursing. Furthermore, these influences and their games of truth cannot account for nursing. The knowledges of nursing itself are to be found in practising nursing, reflecting on it, and coming to understand ways of being which inhere in the relationships between nurse, patient and contexts in which nursing occurs. Inevitably, these knowledges will be grounded in, and will, to a large extent, need to be understood as, complex gestalts, which are temporally, environmentally and ontologically sensitive. They also will be narratives, and they will allow for expressive and meaningful engagement and contact among humans, in both physical and interpersonal senses.

NOTES

1   I use the term in the plural to heighten our understandings of the multiplicities of nursing's ways of knowing. To refer to knowledge in its singular sense is to erroneously suggest that knowledge is some kind of homogenous stuff.

2   This is often the case in mental health nursing; although the problem is non-physical in the sense that we understand illnesses of the object body, many of the issues that concern people with mental illnesses are embodied, for example, feeling depressed and unable to get out of bed and face the day. Self-mutilation and self-abuse are also examples of ways in which the embodied self is caught up with states that we call mental illness.

3   A good example is knowledge about early mobility in the case of serious illness(es); within decades, nursing and medical practices have altered dramatically as concepts about the relative merits of mobility and immobility have been challenged and changed.

4   The most robust knowledge is that which is borne primarily of experience and practising, but which has, necessarily, a cognitive component. For example, one's knowledge of riding a bicycle or making a bed does not deteriorate with age; one's physical prowess, speed, and ability to perform may deteriorate, but the knowledge embedded in performed knowing may not.

5   The authors state, however, that the validity of the Eating Attitude Tests are of 'limited relevance' because their validity for Africans is uncertain.

6   Like many of my colleagues, I have been instructed by reviewers to remove the personal pronoun from research reports and I am sure I am not alone in this experience.

7   Nurses often report that there are events or experiences that they cannot describe in words; this is not to say they are inarticulate, but to indicate the limitations of language as a means of communicating about some events or experiences.

8   Not only is economic discourse inadequate for much of what nursing involves, it is also inappropriate in many circumstances.
9   I would draw a distinction here between some of the discourses of the social sciences, particularly sociology and some aspects of psychology, in which there are attempts to write in the subjective. The dominant theme within these disciplines, however, remains scientific/positivistic and reductive.
10 This term literally means not coping.

REFERENCES

Adverse Drug Reactions Advisory Committee 1994 Australian Adverse Drug Reactions Bulletin 13(1):2–3

Bottorff J L, Varcoe C 1995 Transitions to nurse-patient interactions: a qualitative ethology. Qualitative Health Research, 5(3) 315–313

Brown C, Seddon J 1996 Nurses, doctors and the body of the patient: medical dominance revisited. Nursing Inquiry 3(1)30–35

Bruner J 1990 Acts of meaning. Harvard University Press, Cambridge, Mass.

Cordery C 1995 Doing more with less: nursing and the politics of economic rationalism in the 1990s. In: Gray G, Pratt R Issues in Australasian nursing 4. Churchill Livingstone, Melbourne, 355–374

Coward D D 1990 The lived experience of self-transcendence in women with advanced breast cancer. Nursing Science Quarterly 3(4):162–69

Dennison P D, Keeling A W 1989 Clinical support for eliminating the nursing diagnosis of knowledge deficit. Image: Journal of Nursing Scholarship 21(3):142–144

Dunlop M J 1986 Is a science of caring possible? Journal of Advanced Nursing, 11:661–670

Fahy T A, Robinson P H, Russell G F M, Sheinman B 1988 Anorexia nervosa following torture in a young African woman. British Journal of Psychiatry 153:385–387

Foucault M 1980 Michel Foucault: power/knowledge: selected interviews and other writings, 1972–1977. Harvester press, Brighton

Foucault M 1988 The ethic of care for the self as a practice of freedom. An interview with Michel Foucault. In: Bernauer J, Rasmussen D (eds) The final Foucault. MIT Press, Cambridge, Mass

Grosz E, Probyn E 1996 Sexy bodies: the strange carnalities of feminism. Routledge, London

Jenny J L 1987 Knowledge deficit: not a nursing diagnosis. Image: Journal of Nursing Scholarship 19(4):184–185

Kleinman A 1988 The illness narratives. Suffering, healing and the human condition. Basic Books, New York

Lawler J 1990 The body, dirty work and nursing: toward understanding the invisibility of nursing care. Proceedings of XII Annual Conference of the Royal College of Nursing, Australia, Sydney, 216–229

Lawler J 1991a What you see is not always what you get: seeing, feeling and researching nursing. Proceedings of Nursing research: pro-active vs reactive, Centre for Nursing Research & Royal College of Nursing, Australia, Adelaide, 13–21

Lawler J 1991b Behind the screens: nursing, somology, and the problem of the body. Churchill Livingstone, Melbourne

Lawler J 1991c In search of an Australian identity. In: Gray G, Pratt R (eds) Towards a discipline of nursing. Churchill Livingstone, Melbourne, 211–227

Lawler J 1993 Researching nursing: minding our language and finding our way(s). Proceedings of Research in nursing: turning points, Centre for Nursing Research, Adelaide, 1–11

Lawler J 1994 A study of adult patients' expectations of nurses and the nursing service: some surprises and issues. Proceedings of the Institute of Nurse Administrators of NSW and ACT Conference, Sydney

Little M 1995 Humane medicine, Cambridge University Press, London

Marck P 1990 Therapeutic reciprocity: a caring phenomenon. Advances in Nursing Science 13(1):49–59

Mitchell G J 1991 Nursing diagnosis: an ethical analysis. Image: Journal of Nursing Scholarship 23(2):99–103

Mitchell G J, Santopinto M 1988 An alternative to nursing diagnosis. The Canadian Nurse 84(10):25–28

Moore T 1991 Cry of the damaged man. Picador, Sydney

Parker J, Gardner G 1992 The silence and the silencing of the nurse's voice: a reading of patient progress notes. Australian Journal of Advanced Nursing 9(2):3–9

Parker J, Gardner G, Wiltshire, J 1992 Handover: the collective narrative of nursing practice. Australian Journal of Advanced Nursing 9(3):31–37

Polkinghorne D E 1988 Narrative knowing and the human sciences. State University of New York Press, New York

Reeve T 1993 Coherent & consistent quality assurance & utilisation review activities in public and private hospitals in Australia. Casemix Development Programme, Canberra

Shields D 1978 Nursing care in labour and patient satisfaction: a descriptive study. Journal of Advanced Nursing 3:535–550

Taylor B J 1990 Conservation of natural resources: save ordinariness in nursing. Proceedings of XII Annual Conference of the Royal College of Nursing, Australia, Sydney, 230–249

Taylor B J 1994 Being human. Churchill Livingstone, Melbourne

The Macquarie Dictionary 1991 Macquarie University, Sydney

Van Manen 1990 Researching lived experience, State University of New York, New York

Vincent K G, Coler M S 1990 A unified nursing diagnostic model. Image: Journal of Nursing Scholarship 22(2):93–95

Wortmann C B, Silver R C 1989 The myths of coping with loss. Journal of Consulting and Clinical Psychology 57(3)349–357

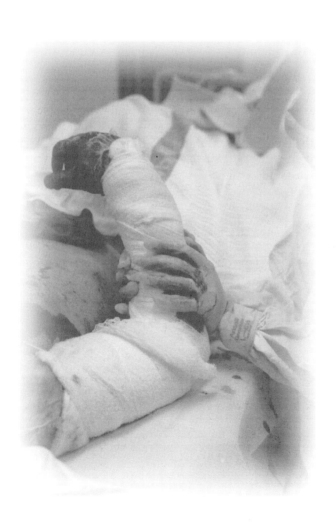

5

The body in health, illness and pain

Irena Madjar

Introduction

In a footnote to her poem 'Understand, old one', Australian poet Oodgeroo of the tribe Noonuccal (formerly known as Kath Walker) sketches the scene which inspired the writing of the verses. She was invited by some 'university people' to an ancient Aboriginal burial ground near Brisbane to witness the exhumation of skeletal remains. Clearly, her experience of the occasion was different from how others, there for a different reason, may have perceived the project which brought them together. The first two stanzas of the poem read:

Understand, old one,
I mean no desecration
Staring here with the learned ones
At your opened grave.
Now after hundreds of years gone
The men of science coming with
*   spade and knowledge*
Peer and probe, handle the yellow bones,
To them specimens, to me
More. Deeply moved am I.

Understand, old one,
I mean no lack of reverence.
It is with love
I think of you so long ago laid here
With tears and wailing.
Strongly I feel your presence very near
Haunting the old spot, watching
As we disturb your bones. Poor ghost,
I know, I know you will understand.

(Oodgeroo of the tribe Noonuccal, formerly Kath Walker 1990:100)

What the poet captures here in such wonderfully evocative language is the contrasting ways of relating to the human body, albeit the posthumous body. For the scientists the bones are specimens, holding secrets about history and likely to yield information about the lifestyle, nutrition and diseases of an earlier era. For the poet, the bones are more personal, connecting her to her own history, and leading her to reflect in the rest of the poem on the time that separates yet cannot 'estrange' the ties that bind her to 'the old one' and the two of them to the people of whom they are an inseparable part.

The ways that we as nurses view, perceive, experience and relate to the human body may be many and varied, yet often in the busyness of the classroom or clinical situation we may not stop to reflect on the taken-for-granted ways in which issues of embodiment are dealt with in nursing practice. We juggle the perspectives of anatomical-physiological understandings with the realities of working with individual persons who laugh, cry, hurt, worry; feel anxious, depressed, contented, happy, frustrated, angry, exhilarated or despondent; and have needs which we, as nurses, often cannot meet or resolve. The nature of modern nursing practice may also focus our attentions on the patient's specific emotional or behavioural responses and on the observable and measurable indicators of the onset, progression, deterioration, recovery, and outcomes of illness. In such a context, the lived, embodied experience of the person is in danger of being overlooked. What is it like to live through sudden, painful trauma such as burns, or to face months of chemotherapy necessitated by a diagnosis of cancer? What do we know of the person's experience when we identify or apply the diagnosis of pain?

In this chapter then, my intention is to explore the nature of human embodiment in the context of illness and particularly of pain. The rather more brief discussion of the body in health, at the beginning of the chapter, will serve only as a starting point and the ground against which to set the ensuing discussion. In my writing I have drawn from a variety of literature sources, including historical, phenomenological, and more recent, sociological literature on *the body*, on my own experiences and reflections as a nurse, but primarily on a research project on the lived experience of clinically inflicted pain conducted as part of my doctoral studies (Madjar 1991).

The body in health

The healthy human body has been variously represented, and at times celebrated throughout human history. From ancient times, sculpture and painting have provided a means of representing the beauty of the human form and the ability of the human body to excel in movement, such as is evident in the cave drawings of hunting scenes or the classical Greek sculptures of young men engaged in sports, or to carry within it the powers of fecundity and procreation. The scientific interest in the human body over the past few centuries, coupled with the development of the scientific method of observation, analysis, and hypothesis-testing, has tended toward a very different view of human embodiment. The material body increasingly came to be seen as an object, separate from the person embodying it, and legitimately the province of anatomical, physiological and molecular levels of inquiry. In nursing and medicine, the emphasis until quite recently was placed on the diseased, malfunctioning, damaged, or in some other way, inadequate body. The healthy body, for the large part was left to the sports trainers, dance teachers, and fashion designers to define, mould, and present for public approval and emulation. The current interest in the body, as it is lived and experienced in everyday life, owes much to phenomenology and especially to early phenomenological writers such as Heidegger (1962), Marcel (1960, 1984), and Merleau-Ponty (1962).

From a phenomenological perspective, the body is our basic mode of being in the world; consciousness is embodied consciousness, and a person is an embodied being, not just a possessor of a body (Merleau-Ponty 1962). The body, 'the incarnate being', is the 'touchstone of existence' and therefore the starting point in the quest for understanding of human experience (Straus & Machado 1984). This distinguishes the lived body from other objects, recognising that there is an inherent uniqueness in how people experience their own bodies for themselves which is different from how they experience external objects. The inborn skills and bodily comportments combine with socially and culturally acquired postures, gestures and habits which give the lived body its unique qualities and a way of being in the world which is uniquely personal.

In health, we experience our embodied selves in an unselfconscious way, taking for granted and paying little attention to processes such as breathing, or the position of each limb in relation to the rest of the body. Based on a study conducted in France during the 1960s, Claudine Herzlich (1973:53) has argued that for many people health is experienced as an 'unawareness of the body', or as 'organic silence'. This idea of the body unaware of itself, of not paying attention to its inner workings, is explored at length by Drew Leder in his 1990 book *The absent body*. He argues that our involvement in the world turns our attention outwards, to the project at hand, whether this be reading or engaging in fierce sporting competition. In such instances one may be 'lost in thought', or completely focused on anticipating the opponent's next move, rather than dwelling on one's own embodiment. The point is that when our being in the world is smooth and effortless, we tend not to be consciously aware of our bodies. It is only when effort is required, such as in climbing a steep hill, or there is a breakdown due to illness or injury, that we become aware of the complex nature of coordinated movement, or the effort involved in breathing and other bodily activities (Sacks 1984, Benner & Wrubel 1989).

Yet, paradoxically, there is at another level a growing interest in the subject of embodiment as seen in the recent sociological literature (Turner 1992, Fox 1993, Scott & Morgan 1993, Shilling 1993), as well as inescapable evidence, particularly in the more affluent societies, of the attention and effort devoted to constructing 'healthy' bodies, through diet, exercise and other self-care activities. Some of the sociological writing, particularly that of Bryan Turner, focuses on the body in health and illness and the way others, including the health professionals, handle the issues of embodiment. Other writers have focused on a variety of issues including, inter alia, gender identities in 'disciplining' the body through exercise (Mansfield & McGinn 1993, Morgan 1993), and mothers' constructions of 'managing' their infants' bodies and keeping them clean (Murcott 1993), which have less to do with matters of health and illness, and more with issues of socially desirable and acceptable presentations of self to others.

The particular relevance of sociological writing in the area of embodiment lies in the contribution such writing can make to our understanding of the social and historical constructions of what count as healthy, fit, attractive, and desirable bodies. Furthermore, sociological and feminist analyses have also highlighted the ways in which medical interventions such as cosmetic surgery or gastric stapling can be seen as having less to do with correcting bodily defects and more with creating appearances which are seen to satisfy social notions of youthfulness, femininity and masculinity (Shilling 1993).

The body in illness

To understand the embodied nature of pain experience, it is necessary to first give some attention to the embodied nature of the experience of illness. While pain may occur in situations other than illness, such as dental treatment or a minor injury, pain often acts as a warning signal of impending tissue damage, such as in myocardial infarction or acute appendicitis; as an indicator of ongoing pathological changes, such as in peripheral vascular disease or the development of neoplastic metastases; as a sign of complications, such as in the development of post-operative peritonitis, or as a persistent symptom which becomes an illness in its own right, such as in the case of chronic back pain. What illness and pain often have in common is their capacity to call forth the awareness of the body, hitherto ignored, taken for granted, and simply lived. It is only when our gaze is turned away from the world and the activities which connect us to the world, and toward ourselves, that we become consciously aware of the effort involved in the usually taken-for-granted bodily activities. Illness and pain (among other experiences) provide the stimulus for such turning toward ourselves, and our increased sensitivity to the functional performance of the body and how the body appears to ourselves and to others (Roy 1976, Roberts 1978, Leder 1984, 1990, Leonard 1994).

Within the Cartesian paradigm of embodiment, the body is apprehended as an object, a machine able to be understood by close scrutiny and mathematical analysis, as any other object may be known (Descartes 1637/ 1986, Campbell 1984, Leder 1984). To conceive of the human body as a physical object with measurable properties of mass, weight, size and motion in relation to other objects, is to provide only a partial account of its characteristics and activity (Madjar 1991). Such a view has made possible the many advances in biomedicine and is clearly of crucial importance in the continuing search for more effective medications and surgical interventions. In this context, the perspective is both valid and justified. To suggest, however, that the human body is no more than 'the assemblage of flesh, bones, and organs which the anatomist anatomizes' and 'what the undertakers bury when they bury you' (Campbell 1984:2), is to ignore the embodied intelligence and skills that connect human beings with the world and allow us to inhabit it in a unique way. While disease affects the anatomical body, it is the person who experiences illness, who suffers, and whose embodiment is affected by bodily changes which go beyond the organic level. In his argument for a phenomenological view of embodiment and human action, Merleau-Ponty (1962) does not reject the presence of the material, anatomical body, understood through 'mechanistic physiology' and able to be seen as a mere physical object. His argument is that the *res extensa*, the object-body of Descartes, is itself a derivative, arising out of the experience of the lived body (Leder 1984). It is also a constructed representation which we take up or ignore depending on the situation and our place in it. Objectification, which dominates delivery of health care services through diagnostic labelling, categorisation, classification, protocols and regulations, encourages nurses and other health care workers to focus on the observable and measurable aspects of illness and to ignore its largely subjective and embodied nature (Gadow 1989). In the process, it is not only the patient, but also the nurse who is objectified and alienated from her or his sense of embodied self, no more dramatically than in the context of clinically inflicted pain (Gadow 1989, Madjar 1991), a topic to be explored further in the latter part of this chapter.

What illness entails above all else is an awareness of changes in one's-being-in-the-world. The familiar 'feeling myself' is lost and needs to be regained. Others have written about different ways in which the human body has been constructed by nurses, as obedient, sinful, sanitised, stigmatised, dangerous, desexualised, deceitful, and communicating (Hickson & Holmes 1994). Each of these constructions deserves deeper exploration. My focus for the remainder of the chapter, however, will be not on how others construct their bodies or their illnesses, but on the patients' own lived experiences of illness and pain and the themes that arose out of the study with patients receiving intravenous chemotherapy for cancer and patients in a burn care unit (Madjar 1991).

Losing the habitual body

The habitual body for many of us is the body we live and know from inside ourselves, the body we take for granted, the body which is upstanding and reliable, the body that sleeps at night and wakes in the morning, the body that moves effortlessly and without our consciously willing it to do so. It is the loss of this familiar body that signals illness, and a deep-seated, embodied need to regain the familiar sense of the habitual body, or as people often express it — to be oneself again.

The loss of the familiar body often begins with sensing that *something is wrong*. Whether suddenly, as in the case of burn injuries, or slowly and sometimes insidiously as in those who develop cancer, there is a breakdown, a sense of discontinuity with the world which has lost its predictability, and its responsiveness to the person. Where there was smooth skin and soft tissue before, there is now a palpable lump in the breast — a small but frightening focus for doubt and fear. Once felt, it cannot be not felt. The taken-for-granted reliability of the body is shattered as surely as it may be shattered by sudden burn trauma as hot wax accidentally pours down a woman's arm, or a driver fights the flames as he pushes his way out of a burning truck.

The loss of the familiar body is further accentuated by the awareness of *looking different to oneself and to the world*. For patients with cancer this may come slowly as the effects of disease and chemotherapy gradually take their toll and they lose not only weight and sometimes hair, but also the sparkle in the eye and the springiness in their step. For those with burn injuries, coming to terms with a strange, disfigured, hurting body may be more confronting and often extremely difficult. A young woman whose face and head were burned, after seeing herself in the mirror for the first time, expressed her struggle in the following words:

Patient: *I try and put a patch on it. I try and imagine that it's not there, or it's not really as bad as it looks. ...I don't really feel that this is part of my body in a way. This is something else and Geraldine will be Geraldine as she was on Friday, in a few weeks.*

Researcher: *But this is not Geraldine?*

Patient: *No! No, this is another body.*

Researcher: *Another body?*

Patient: *Mm. This is another body that I don't know. Not me. I don't deserve it. It's not me. I don't deserve it. I've been saying that to myself all day. And I was hoping that it will go away. (Madjar 1991:120–121)*

Several weeks later as this woman continued to struggle to come to terms with her injuries, the sense of alienation from her own disfigured body and the loss of the person she had been was still very much in evidence:

Patient: *I think I would have been quite happy with all the grafting on my body, except my head. I think to lose my hair has been quite upsetting   for me... I liked my hair. I looked in the mirror today...and I thought I looked like something from outer space. I knew I would see myself like that. It's just a little too soon yet.*

Researcher: *What do you see when you look in the mirror?*

Patient: *A ruined face...half of it anyway, and it makes me feel very angry...I'd really like to get back into my life and forget what happened, and that's impossible. ...It's not as though I am going to walk out of here with a face that's exactly like it was before. I can see that now. It's not going to be the same. There are going to be differences, and people are going to notice differences...I think that I will feel very, very vulnerable out in the open.*

The [left] hand has never been anything great for me to look at. I've never really been able to pick it up and say 'Doesn't it look wonderful?' or, 'Isn't that looking better?' At the moment it's pretty horrible.

Researcher: *What does it feel like?*

Patient: *It feels like an old woman's hand, and it looks like about a ninety-year old woman's hand. ...It does not look like mine. I look at this [injured, left] hand here, and then I look at that one [uninjured, right], they are not the same at all. ...In a funny sort of way I can't really see myself as myself again. Not really. I think I've got a long way to go before that happens. (Madjar 1991:121–122)*

Loss of the familiar body comes not only through looking different but also through *feeling different* . For people with cancer, this *feeling different* may start with the diagnosis and intensify as they undergo diagnostic procedures and commence medical treatment. The struggle for these people is to submit to therapy which has the power to make them feel uncomfortable, depressed, and different, and can trap them into a situation in which they feel they have no choice and no control. Like patients with burns, patients with cancer may come to understand that their lives can be lived only through the ailing bodies from which they cannot escape. The following interview excerpt comes from a middle-aged man, describing what it feels like to have chronic leukaemia:

My feeling generally about it is that I've caught something. It's a virus thing that starts it apparently. ...It's done its damage and I am stuck with this body and what is going on in it and is going to have to go on. ...

My glands come up over here, under the chin, and that's fairly noticeable. They get really quite large. They are uncomfortable. ...I feel confused. Oh, I feel hopeless about it sometimes. I know I can't get away from it. ...I think it's a feeling of being trapped; you know you are trapped, but then, that's life. (Madjar 1991:123–124)

For some patients the illness and the medical treatment may be imbued with powers which can alienate them from their own bodies and reduce them to a position of a helpless onlooker in a battle between the disease which has taken over the body and the therapy which aims to destroy, or at least control the disease. A man in his 30s, a fit and healthy sportsman until diagnosed with cancer, described his once familiar body as a battlefield, with cancer and medicine the two opposing forces, and he himself a mere spectator:

Patient: *The cancer is either going to control me, or the medicine is going to control me, and apart from doing what I am told, and my diet, and things like that, I don't think that there is anything personally that I can do. Either the cancer is going to win, or the medicine is going to win. I don't know.*

Researcher: *Where does that leave you?*

Patient: *It leaves me with a real horrible feeling in that I don't know which is going to win. I know which one I want! ...It's either going to be the medicine or the cancer that wins, and there is not a lot I can do. (Madjar 1991:127–128)*

For some people, the illness or injuries are such that they *feel overwhelmed*, unable to see beyond their present situation or to project themselves into a different and more optimistic future. Their 'embodied knowledge', of sensing from inside oneself, may not be balanced or integrated with other forms of knowing such as the 'conscious, cognitive knowing', based on information from medical and other sources, and 'socially shared knowing' which comes from culturally developed meanings, in this case, of illness (Gordon 1990:276). The embodied knowing of one's own illness can be powerful in demonstrating the facticity of our corporeal existence (Merleau-Ponty 1962), and the frailty and finitude of the only body through which each of us is able to live a life. While the physical body may be repaired, or the disease arrested and brought under control, the person may remain caught in the web of illness and unable to move beyond it.

Regaining the habitual body and becoming oneself again

For some patients this sense of looking, feeling and being different, of not being themselves, may be persistent and overwhelming. Some cannot see a way out. *Regaining the habitual body and becoming oneself again* requires that patients see themselves as moving toward a better future, rather than remaining trapped in their present, or wishing for a magical return to a happier past. For some, regaining their sense of embodiment may be an exciting and almost joyous experience as they resume the temporary interruption to the flow of life. In the following interview excerpt there is an almost palpable sense of joy as the woman talks of drawing back to herself her badly burned arm which only a few days earlier had felt alien and strange:

Patient: *I felt glad that she [nurse] was cutting it off [debriding dead skin], and I could see the smooth skin again underneath. ...I suppose it's a good feeling to know that underneath the dead skin there is life again; there is new skin again underneath. ...You are reliant upon someone else to do what they can for you.*

Researcher: *How does that feel?*

Patient: *I don't know how to answer that, ...but I know it wasn't me, it wasn't my body. I felt as if I was getting help from other people to give me back what was mine before all this happened. I suppose your body has been through a big shock. Your body has to readjust. I was glad for the physiotherapist coming in to give me back movement in my fingers to start off with. It was really quite sore while she worked on it. And then she worked on my wrist and I felt 'oh good, something's coming back'. And she actually got on to my elbow, and I felt 'hurrah, I've got my arm back!' You do feel as if you've lost part of your body, and you rely on others to give it back to you. (Madjar 1991:136)*

For other patients the *regaining of a sense of being oneself* may be much more difficult. They may not be able to resume their lives where they had left off when interrupted by injury or illness. Regaining the habitual body and becoming oneself again may be experienced as an impossible task, so that the only way forward has to involve the *creation of a new kind of future,* and a constitution of self as a changed person, perhaps one with a reduced life expectancy or a different outlook.

For still others the challenge may be to *live through each round* of uncomfortable or painful treatment while the rest of their life remains in limbo. Being oneself is a temporary achievement which lasts only until the next treatment round approaches. A major issue for some patients in the study (Madjar 1991) was the *fighting to remain a person*, rather than allowing themselves to become totally passive and powerless observers of their wounded bodies. They felt able to endure the pain and the discomforts of their illness and injuries, but not the passive acquiescence frequently required of them. They accepted their treatments as necessary and bearable but did not see them as the only means through which their bodies would heal. The essential part of being able to become themselves again was their ability to draw on others' support and on their own personal and spiritual resources, and on being able to assert themselves through their own choices and actions. In the following interview excerpt, the woman in her late 30s makes it very clear that her vegetarian diet is not used in the expectation of a miracle cure, rather it is a means of asserting her strong need to be actively involved in the healing process:

> I am eating a hundred per cent raw (vegetarian) diet at the moment and I really feel good in myself. Whether it does me any good or not, I feel good because I am doing something for myself. Something that I feel is going to be helpful. ...That's the big thing, the thought that I am doing something for myself. I don't want to just sit back and let people be doing things to me. ...I want to get better and there's things I want to do. I want to go back to work and get some money, take trips overseas. So I'd rather aim for that and I know it mightn't work out that way, but at least I am trying and it makes me feel so much better, the knowing that I am trying. (Madjar 1991:139)

There were also some patients in the study who felt so changed and overwhelmed by their experience that they could not envisage themselves as themselves again. They felt alienated and even repulsed by their bodies, regarded their bodies as uncooperative (for example, when they would *not behave themselves* and yield blood samples easily), or as hostile entities that would not let them rest or sleep. They felt let down by bodies that could no longer be relied on to look and feel normal, and they felt trapped within the bodies and situations that they wished to leave but realised they could not. As one person expressed it, rather wistfully: 'The trouble is, I can have only this body and that's it'.

It is worth noting that the outcome of the struggle to *regain their habitual bodies and become themselves again* did not depend on the extent of the patients' injuries or their chances of cancer remission with chemotherapy. In other words, 'objectively' defined risks to survival and recovery did not determine their sense of being whole and themselves again. Rather, how far they travelled was influenced by their capacity to see beyond the confines of their present situation and to project themselves into a personal future with a degree of hope and optimism. This is in no way to suggest that recovery is a question of mind over matter. Hope, too, is an embodied experience and one lived in the context of availability of, and accessibility to, effective treatments, and the socially shared knowledge about the likely outcomes of illness, or what Good (cited in Gordon 1990:277) has called 'the political economy of hope'. To discuss illness as an embodied experience is not to be confined to the purely subjective and idiosyncratic; it is rather to recognise the extent to which people constitute and are in turn constituted by their experiences of illness and of their being in the world (Benner & Wrubel 1989, Madjar 1991).

The body in pain

For those who experience it, pain is not an objective, measurable entity, as it might appear in the scientific literature. Rather, pain has the capacity to enter the very fabric of one's body and to destroy the familiar, taken-for-granted being in the world. There is no bodily silence or absence in pain. Addis (1986) suggests that pain imposes its presence, requiring that one attend to it, not only by its intensity but also, as Merleau-Ponty (1962) too has indicated, by its spatiality — it is always located in a certain place in the body.

In her philosophical exploration on the vulnerability of the human body and the political consequences of deliberately inflicted pain, Elaine Scarry (1985) identifies some of the essential qualities of pain as its *invisibility* and its *inexplicability*, making it possible for a person to be physically near someone in pain and not be aware of that pain. Unlike other states of consciousness, bodily pain has no outside point of reference, no referential content. It just is. 'It is not *of* or *for* anything. It is precisely because it takes no object that it, more than any other phenomenon, resists objectification in language' (Scarry 1985:5). Our vocabulary is not equal to the task of communicating bodily pain. In the words of Virginia Woolf (1967:194):

> English, which can express the thoughts of Hamlet and the tragedy of Lear has no words for the shiver or the headache...The merest schoolgirl when she falls in love has Shakespeare or Keats to speak her mind for her, but let a sufferer try to describe a pain in his head to a doctor and language at once runs dry.

Marcel (1984:335) also speaks of the 'uncommunicable aspect' of pain which may contribute to the feelings of not only being threatened, but also of being trapped in a hurting body which has taken on the role of a master. The pain, too, can become a tormentor, calling attention to itself and robbing the person of rest and sleep. Describing his experience of pain associated with herpes zoster, T H White, wrote in his diary, quoted by his biographer:

> The pain of shingles is a penetrating or convecting mixture of aches or soreness. It is a nagging pain, not noble like kidney stone or leaping like a beating ... but petty and altering and unrelenting though moving from one situation to another, like a woman scolding all night. ...Kidney stone is a steady, quiet Colossus — you can almost love him, certainly give him

homage and respect. Fire, cane, touched-tooth nerves and others certainly make you jump to attention. They are great as far as that goes, at all events they have authority. But this bloody ceaseless shingles is a petty torturer who goes from here to there with mean variations, never a great tyrant or ruler, but a hired assistant (3rd murderer in plays) who slinks about with ceaseless, varying, mean repertoire of torments. Stab? yes. Ache? yes. Even itch. And he goes on all night. (Warner 1967:297)

Those who, like T H White, have written about their experiences have done so most often by resorting to metaphors in which pain is personified and presented as something external to oneself. Thus one can 'talk' *to* one's pain even as one is unable to talk *about* it to others. At the same time, the metaphors act to obscure our inability to describe the pain itself in its embodied existence, and our need to present it as something other (a nagging woman, a petty torturer, a stab, an itch) which invite the listener to apprehend the experience in more understandable terms. Thus, because bodily pain resists objectification in language, it is marked by a strong element of *unshareability*. In other words, pain silences and actively destroys language, one of the culturally learned ways of being in the world with others. Furthermore, the reversion to a prelanguage state of cries and moans also signifies the destruction of the person's habitual body, no longer able to express its anguish in ways that others can fully comprehend. The situation is compounded by the health professionals unable or unwilling to hear patients' expressions of pain. In Scarry's words (1985:6–7), they may:

> ...perceive the voice of the patient as an 'unreliable narrator' of bodily events, a voice which must be by-passed as quickly as possible so that they can get around and behind it to the physical events themselves. But if the only external sign of the felt-experience of pain...is the patient's verbal report... then to by-pass the voice is to by-pass the bodily event, to by-pass the patient, to by-pass the person in pain.

Most importantly, perhaps, the subjectivity of pain makes it into something that cannot be either confirmed or denied. It is precisely because we know our own bodies in a way that is fundamentally different from the way we know anyone else's body that '...to have pain is to have *certainty*; to hear about pain is to have *doubt*.' (Scarry 1985:13). Yet for the patients who experience pain there is no doubt about the reality and the painfulness of their pain. When, however, health professionals question and doubt the reported experience, they often add to the suffering of the person in pain.

The nature of clinically inflicted pain

Clinically inflicted pain may be one of the most frequently overlooked aspects of the patients' experiences of illness and medical and nursing care. The term is used here to refer to *any pain experienced by patients that is directly attributable to procedures or tasks performed on them by health care workers.* More specifically, it includes pain associated with procedures during which the person's body is touched, handled, invaded by instruments such as needles, or where body tissue is removed, for example, in taking of biopsies or removal of dead or infected tissue in the process of skin debridement. The context of such pain is not so much the physical world of the hospital, or the social world of family, hospital staff, or other patients. For the patients, the most intimate context for their experience of pain are the changes in the embodied self resulting from disease or injury. The changes brought about by illness or trauma relate to pain in at least two different ways.

First, bodily changes brought about by tissue trauma and disease pathology *predicate* pain since without them pain would not occur, and there would be no need for diagnostic and treatment procedures that give rise to inflicted pain. Second, bodily changes also *situate pain* into a body which is not the normal, familiar body the person knows and through which he or she knows the world. From a situation in which the body is taken for granted, ignored in terms of its anatomical structures, and simply lived, the patient with cancer or burn injuries is placed in a situation of acute awareness of a body which is a source of worrying and unpleasant sensations, which does not behave in predictable ways, which is no longer reliable, and which may threaten one's very existence. It is in this context that patients experience further assaults on their bodily integrity through experiences of disease-related as well as clinically inflicted pain.

To understand inflicted pain as a lived rather than as an observed, and therefore objective, experience it is necessary to turn to the thing itself — the immediate, prereflective awareness of life or in this case, life in pain. The lived experience provides the starting point for the project of describing the phenomenon. For the patient with burn injuries, for example, the observed experience and that recorded in nursing notes is one of saline baths, debridement of dead tissue, grafting of new skin, and dressing changes. But the lived experience evident in patients' narratives is of *hurt and painfulness* of inflicted pain, of its *wounding* nature, of the ongoing need to *hand one's body over* to others to treat and to wound, and of the pressures to *restrain the body and the voice* when in pain, in order to retain composure and make easier the work of others. These then are the four essential themes that describe the phenomenon of clinically inflicted pain.

The hurt and painfulness of inflicted pain

Perhaps the most obvious, and yet the most likely to be overlooked, quality of inflicted pain is its sheer *painfulness*. Such pain is much more than an unpleasant sensation. It hurts and it has an immediacy of bodily presence which makes it difficult to ignore and at the same time, in this embodied sense, impossible to share with others. It is this unshareability of the essential painfulness of pain that creates a gulf between those who feel the pain but cannot relieve it, and those who, despite personal contribution to its genesis, cannot feel it, yet retain control over the means of its amelioration and relief. For those whose work involves the performance of invasive and painful procedures, the report of inflicted pain invites doubt as to its presence and intensity.

The lived experience of the person on whom pain is inflicted is not one of doubt, but of certainty of the inescapable presence of pain within a wounded, hurting body. The embodied nature of the painfulness of pain is experienced as different from discomforts inherent in restricted movements or the need to maintain a particular posture. In the patients' lived experience it is also different from the dis-ease of anxiety, the dread of anticipation, or the fear of mutilation, even though all of these may be present at the same time as pain. Thus, while nurses may doubt another's pain, interpreting it as anxiety, fear, or inability to behave like a mature adult, patients on whom pain is inflicted know through their bodies the essential *hurt* and *painfulness* of pain.

The wounding nature of inflicted pain

While the hurt and painfulness is an essential quality of all pain, one of the things which sets inflicted pain apart from pathological pain resulting from disease is the *wounding* nature of inflicted pain. It is not only that the invasive procedures which puncture, pierce, cut, or tear living tissue are themselves wounding, but more specifically, that pain resulting from such procedures is also wounding. The body already marred by disease such as cancer or the trauma of burn injuries, and in the latter case already in pain, is further wounded in the course of diagnostic and treatment procedures. For people who have lost a sense of bodily integrity, new attacks on the body bring pain and feelings of being exposed and vulnerable to further wounding and further pain.

The observed experience may be of a person having blood drawn for laboratory analysis, or undergoing a change of dressings. The lived experience is one of *wounding* and *vulnerability*, and almost always, of pain. The observed experience involves medical instruments being used to accomplish a necessary task, but the lived experience is of *weapons* — invading, poking and jabbing, 'digging around' and 'harpooning' the body which offers no protection and no escape. In the words of one patient describing his experience of a femoral artery puncture:

> They can fish around there, and I say 'fish' literally. It should be 'harpooning' because if they don't get the thing straight away they just keep jabbing and poking. ...There's got to be a better way to take [blood] gas samples than digging around. ...The last one took twenty minutes and you just have to lie there as though it isn't happening to you. (Madjar 1991:160)

The *wounding* nature of inflicted pain is evident in the strong and unequivocal language used to describe the lived experience. The language is a poignant record of the pre-reflective, raw experience of pain that 'burns', 'sears', 'stings' and 'hurts' in a 'horrible', 'excruciating', 'exhausting', 'distressing', and sometimes 'overwhelming' way (see Table 5.1).

Table 5.1 Descriptive terms related to inflicted pain used by patients with burns

Sensory	Evaluative	Affective
burning	awful	crying
stinging	bad	frightening
searing	endless	distressing
sharp	horrible	tiring
sore	excruciating	exhausting
hurting	powerful	revolting
tender	unbearable	
pinching	overwhelming	
	extreme	

This is the language of forceful metaphors, trying to make visible the invisible, and to share the unshareable. People in pain, whether writers such as T H White cited earlier, or any others hoping to have their pain relieved, depend on such language being heard, on being able to communicate clearly and unambiguously the nature of their experience, and on engaging others in the task of relieving the pain. Metaphorical language serves as a means of having the lived experience of *wounding* 'lifted into the visible world' (Scarry 1985); a means of making the experience matter to others, especially those able to stop the wounding and relieve the pain.

Handing one's body over to others

Whatever its origin, all pain is characterised by hurt and painfulness. This, then, is its first and the most pervasive characteristic. The second one, as just summarised, is the essentially wounding nature of pain, which stands out in relation to inflicted pain, but is not necessarily limited to it.

A further integral feature of clinically inflicted pain in adults is the patient's consent to, and involvement in, the generation of such pain. The pains of physical assault, torture, or self-harm have the qualities of painfulness and wounding, but they do not typically require that the person willingly *hand over his or her body to others* to hurt and to wound. In the clinical context, however, this is an essential component which makes possible the infliction of pain, and sets limits on how the person in pain can act in the situation and cope with the pain.

The essence of clinically inflicted pain is not only that *the pain hurts me*, or that *the actions of another hurt me*, but that *I invite the pain by making my body available to another to wound and to hurt*. Handing one's body over to others is not a passive process of acquiescence. Rather, it requires that patients allow others free access to their bodies, knowing that such access is likely to result in pain, while at the same time keeping sufficient control over their bodies to retain outward composure and not hinder others' work. The lived body, with its intentionality, can facilitate others' work, or it can act as an obstacle, frustrating such work and making pain more likely. Thus, while it is the actions of another which inflict the pain, the patient is not a passive bystander to the event of pain generation. It is not only that he or she must endure the pain, but that in presenting a marred, damaged, uncooperative, or in some other way inadequate body, the person becomes implicated in the generation of pain.

The body which has lost its integrity through illness is more *woundable* and open to the possibility of pain. For example, the patient with cancer who presents an arm swollen with lymphoedema, or veins made fragile by past exposures to chemotherapy, is made aware of an inadequate body which itself must bear some of the responsibility for the pain inflicted on it. Hence clinically inflicted pain involves not only another's actions on *my* body but also *my* inability to present an adequate body which would not impede the work of another. In their communication, nurses may contribute to patients' perceptions of their bodies as inadequate material on which others must work, and thus their perceptions of responsibility for the pain. The following extract from field notes relates to a patient with cancer having his second chemotherapy treatment:

9.50 am

(Nurse attempts to insert an intravenous needle. First attempt unsuccessful.)

Nurse:	*Missed.*
Patient:	*That hurt!* (face becoming slightly flushed, frowns and looks cross)
Nurse:	*Your skin is really tough. I think I just pushed too hard and missed. The outside skin is too hard. Must be all that toughening up from* [playing] *your cricket. ...Do you want me to get someone else?*
Patient:	*No!* (adamant tone of voice and then concerned) *You are not going to give up on me, are you?* (receives no response)
Nurse:	*How much did you have to drink this morning?*
Patient:	*Two cups of coffee.* (again no response from the nurse who spends the next ten minutes silently tapping patient's hand, rubbing it, coaxing a vein almost)
Nurse:	*You are like a cow that won't let down its milk!* (laughs and continues tapping, rubbing, feeling for a vein)
10.02 am	*Needle inserted successfully. (Madjar 1991:158–159)*

Restraining the body and the voice

Part of handing one's body over to others involves retaining adequate control over the body so that it does not impede the work of others. Our habitual being in the world tends toward avoidance of pain and yet, in the clinical situation, this inclination must be overcome and the body restrained so that it remains available to those who must work on it. Furthermore, clinically inflicted pain not only results from actions of others, but much of it must be endured in their presence. The social situation in which clinically inflicted pain must be endured thus creates its own imperatives, including the requirement that the patient behave with composure and cooperation. To do otherwise would not only interfere with the work of others, but would challenge the legitimacy of their actions, as well as the patients' willingness and ability to keep to their side of the implied contract. The patients' work is to endure and to do so in a way that facilitates rather than hampers the work of others, as illustrated in the following account by a young woman remembering a change of dressing on her burned hand:

Patient: *When I first put the hand in Savlon™ [solution], and I actually started undressing, taking the dressing off myself, I didn't really mind that. But when it got down to the part where the hand was quite visible and very painful, then my tolerance level was quite low and I cried...and I felt that I shouldn't be.*

Researcher: Why did you feel that you shouldn't be?

Patient: *It was strange because the nurse said to me 'the injection should be working now, so you shouldn't be feeling any pain'. So I felt guilty when I did feel pain...to a degree. Because the fact is that* **I did feel pain,** *and it was horrible pain. ...I became very tense and very uptight, and I couldn't talk or even cry as I really wanted to.* (Madjar 1991:161)

By *restraining the body and the voice* people in pain exercise a degree of control over themselves and their world. Situated in an unfamiliar, hostile world in which disease and injuries, contingencies of treatment, and the will of others dominate, they need to hold on to that which is still under their control. Thus *restraining one's body and voice* is a means of asserting control over a shrinking sphere of personal influence, in this case one's body (however affected by disease and injuries), and one's communication with the world (however unresponsive that world might be to the person's needs and desires). As already cited, Scarry (1985) reminds us that intense bodily pain is 'language-destroying', deconstructing complex prose into a series of pre-verbal moans, whimpers, and screams. It is a frightening prospect, for to be reduced to this level of being and communication is to lose the dignity and sense of worth inherent in being human; it is to be dehumanised. *Restraining the body and the voice* is thus an essential aspect of enduring clinically inflicted pain and its legitimised wounding and destructiveness. But the experience is more complex than that. When present, *the voice* has the power to influence the shared situation, to force others to take notice; when absent, it allows those who inflict pain to define the situation in their own terms, bypassing the lived experience of the person in pain. Thus, *restraining the body and the voice* is an essential way of being in pain which facilitates the work of others, and allows the person to maintain outward composure, while at the same time adding to the ultimate unshareability of the experience of pain.

Of the four essential themes that describe the nature of clinically inflicted pain (its *hurt and painfulness*, its *wounding nature, handing one's body over to others,* and *restraining the body and the voice*), some are shared with other types of pain, while others are specific to this condition. The *hurt and painfulness* is the essential quality of all pain, regardless of its genesis or circumstances. The quality of *wounding* may be present in different types of pain, but is especially evident in the case of any inflicted pain, whether in the context of clinical treatment, assault, or torture. These two aspects of clinically inflicted pain are inherent in pain being pain, and in the wounding nature of another's actions which create the pain. In other words, the pain has an existence of its own, within the body of the person and yet independent of the person's intentions.

What gives clinically inflicted pain its particular quality is the nature of involvement required of the person on whom pain is inflicted. It is the voluntary nature of the *handing of one's body over to others* to wound and to hurt, and the voluntary (even though also socially expected) efforts to *restrain the body and the voice* from offering resistance or complaint, which distinguish clinically inflicted pain from other forms of inflicted pain. The nature of personal involvement in the clinical situation both invites the pain and cedes control over its duration and intensity to others. Thus *handing one's body over to others* and *restraining the body and the voice* are not incidental to the pain, or merely aspects of the patient role. Rather, they define the nature of the lived experience of clinically inflicted pain in which personal consent and cooperation must be present.

When personal consent and cooperation are withheld, i.e. when the person resists making his or her body available to others and makes no effort to restrain the body and the voice, then the very nature of the situation is changed. This difference makes more comprehensible the distinction which nurses in the study (Madjar 1991) drew between working with adults and working with children, and the stress they experienced when inflicting pain on the latter. Unlike adults, children do not usually voluntarily *hand their bodies over* to be hurt and wounded, and neither do they necessarily *restrain their bodies and their voices* (Offsay 1989). As a result, their bodies may be restrained against their will and, as far as possible, their voices are ignored or the meaning reinterpreted as indicative not of pain but of fear and of inability to grasp the good intent inherent in the actions of others. In such situations nurses may reason that their actions are necessary, therapeutic, and therefore justified, but the patients' behaviour provides forceful evidence of the pain and harm being done to the person. To be permitted at all, restraining of the patient's body against the person's will and persisting with a procedure despite his or her protestations has to be constructed as therapeutic in intent and outcome. The immediate experience, however, is of wounding and pain forced on a person who is not free to refuse them. Such a situation may give rise to the ethical question of the patient's right to refuse treatment where the pain caused against the patient's expressed wishes may be seen as violence, rather than therapy.

Thus, clinically inflicted pain is defined not only by the objective legitimacy of the therapeutic situation, but rather more so by the personal involvement of the patient on whom pain is inflicted. It is the nature of the social situation in which it occurs, and which requires both a therapeutic intent from the person inflicting the pain and active cooperation from the patient, which makes inflicted pain distinctive.

Embodiment, pain, and nursing involvement

The phenomenon of clinically inflicted pain presented here emerged out of the patients' lived experiences. For them, such pain was first and foremost a direct, embodied, elemental experience, grasped as meaningful in terms of its immediate hurt and painfulness. The nurses, on the other hand, did not and could not have direct experience of the patients' pain. Indeed, it is because they do not feel the pain which the patient feels that nurses are able to perform procedures which patients experience as painful. Yet, if the patients' experiences of pain were totally private and inaccessible to nurses, then infliction of pain would not present as a problem, or as a source of stress to nurses. If they were unaware of patients' suffering, then they would not feel the need to shield themselves from it.

The exigencies of treatment bring the nurse and the patient into close physical contact with each other, and it is in this context of a tactile encounter between them that pain comes into being. Yet it is also the tactile encounter that demonstrates their separateness and their very different views of the situation. It is the patient's body which is exposed and open to the gaze of others. The nurse is the one who touches and the patient the one who is touched, but the touch which they share often lacks a quality of empathic intent that would bring them together in a shared understanding of what each is experiencing. Rather, the touch may be instrumental, determined by technical purposes, often breaking through the boundaries of the patient's physical body, penetrating and invading, and bringing pain into the patient's bodily space. The nurse may undress, expose, examine, touch, manipulate, comfort, or hurt the body. She (or he) may treat the body as an object, with distancing and detachment, as a field on which she performs with skill and expertise. Yet, the patient can do none of these. The nurse is hidden away, behind the uniform, the sterile gown, the mask, the gloves. Her (or his) body is inaccessible, even to the extent that the patient may wish to squeeze her (or his) hand in a silent plea for understanding and reassurance.

Nursing education prepares nurses to care, to provide comfort, to ease pain, to relieve suffering. The image we as nurses have of ourselves, and would like others to have of us, does not usually include inflicting pain and discomfort. And yet, the lifeworld of nursing practice, especially in acute care hospitals, includes work which often results in pain. It is a part of nursing practice on which we do not choose to dwell and which we do not feel comfortable debating in public. It is a source of personal unease and stress; it challenges our self perceptions as kind and caring professionals, and points to our inability to eliminate pain and suffering.

Nurses can constitute pain infliction in many different ways. They can regard it as a delegated medical task over which they have no control. It can then become something that is not seen in its own right or as deserving particular attention. It becomes an inseparable part of the treatment procedure during which it is generated, and assumes the same necessity, justification, inevitability, and expected benefits. Subsumed in this way, inflicted pain can easily become invisible. When the patient's body and voice are restrained and the lived experience overlooked, the pain and its impact on the person can be doubted or constructed into something inevitable, non-harmful, and even necessary for recovery. However, as many nurses demonstrate in their daily practice, it is also possible to remain attentive to patients' experiences and mindful of the pain and discomfort nurses' actions can bring. The nurse can relate to the person as a 'lived body', at all times aware of the need to maintain her orientation toward the living person with whom one can form a *therapeutic partnership* (Madjar 1991). The experience of a painful procedure then becomes a shared project; of sharing individual perceptions, of pacing the procedure, of ceding control over how much pain should be endured to the patient, of responding to the situation as it unfolds rather than to an abstract construction of the situation used to justify pain infliction. It is one way in which pain infliction may be openly recognised as an actual part of nurses' work which requires its own particular combination of knowledge, skills, sensitivity, moral commitment, and being in the situation.

Wanting to care and having to inflict discomfort and pain are dissonant and not easily reconcilable facets of nurses' work with patients in many clinical settings. The professional commitment to care and the desire to respond with compassion to a fellow human being is often in conflict with the rational argument inherent in justifying the necessity of inflicting pain in the process of clinical work. This inner dissonance is difficult to sustain and the risk is that the compassionate response will be suppressed, robbing nursing intervention of its human warmth and feeling and thereby dehumanising both the patient and the nurse.

However justifiable the pain we must inflict, we should never forget that all pain hurts. When inflicted with technical detachment and without feeling of regret, pain dehumanises not only the person who must endure it but also the person who inflicts it. There are real dangers in clinical situations in which technological needs supersede nurses' desire to practise 'caring as a moral art', or where 'avoidant strategies interfere with compassionate care, and can cause an emotional numbing that can reach all aspects of the nurse's life' (Benner & Wrubel 198:xi, 377). To inflict pain on a daily basis and train oneself to feel nothing of the other's pain is to be diminished as a person, to compromise one's own sense of wholeness and moral responsibility, and one's commitment to the centrality of caring in nursing practice.

Because nurses experience pain infliction as a difficult and stressful aspect of their work, there is always the temptation to construct it as necessary, as inevitable, as not hurting as much or as long as other kinds of pain, or as non-harmful and even as beneficial to patients' recovery (Madjar 1991). Such constructions mask the essential nature of clinically inflicted pain and its presence as something embodied. The recognition and understanding of the lived, embodied experience of illness and pain, on the other hand, calls for thoughtful, reflective practice which recognises fully its freedom and its responsibility, particularly when engaging in actions that may further hurt those made vulnerable and exposed by illness and need for treatment and professional care.

REFERENCES

Addis L 1986 Pains and other secondary mental entities. Philosophy and Phenomenological Research 47(1):59–73

Benner P, Wrubel J 1989 The primacy of caring: Stress and coping in health and illness. Addison-Wesley, Menlo Park

Campbell K 1984 Body and Mind, 2nd edn. University of Notre Dame Press, Notre Dame

Descartes R 1986 A discourse on method. Meditations and principles. J M Dent & Sons, London (first published in 1637)

Fox N J 1993 Postmodernism, sociology and health. Open University Press, Buckingham

Gadow S 1989 Clinical subjectivity. Advocacy with silent patients. Nursing Clinics of North America 24(2):535–541

Gordon D R 1990 Embodying illness, embodying cancer. Culture, Medicine and Psychiatry 14:275–297

Heidegger M 1962 Being and time. Harper & Row, New York

Herzlich C 1973 Health and Illness: a social psychological analysis. Translated by D Graham. Academic Press, London

Hickson P, Holmes C 1994 Nursing the postmodern body: a touching case. Nursing Inquiry 1:3–14

Leder D 1984 Medicine and paradigms of embodiment. Journal of Medicine and Philosophy 9:29–43

Leder D 1990 The absent body. University of Chicago Press, Chicago

Leonard V W 1994 A Heideggerian phenomenological perspective on the concept of person, In: Benner P (ed) Interpretive phenomenology: embodiment, caring, and ethics in health and illness. Sage, Thousand Oaks

Madjar I 1991 Pain as embodied experience: a phenomenological study of clinically inflicted pain in adult patients. Unpublished PhD thesis. Massey University, New Zealand

Mansfield A, McGinn B 1993 The muscular and the feminine. In: Scott S, Morgan D (eds) Body matters: essays in the sociology of the body. Falmer Press, London, 49–68

Marcel G 1960 Mystery of being. Henry Regnery (Gateway edn), Chicago

Marcel G 1984 Reply to R M Zaner (The mystery of the body-qua-mine). In: Schlipp P A, Hahn L E (eds) The philosophy of Gabriel Marcel. Open Court Publishing, La Salle, 334–335

Merleau-Ponty M 1962 Phenomenology of perception. Translated by C Smith. Routledge & Kegan Paul, New York

Morgan D 1993 You too can have a body like mine: reflections on the male body and masculinities. In: Scott S, Morgan D (eds) Body matters: essays in the sociology of the body. Falmer Press, London, 69–88

Murcott A 1993 Purity and pollution: body management and the social place of infancy. In: Scott S, Morgan D (eds) Body matters: essays in the sociology of the body. Falmer Press, London, 122–134

Offsay J B 1989 The pain of childhood leukaemia: a parent's recollection. Journal of pain and symptom management 4(4):174–178

Oodgeroo Noonuccal (formerly Kath Walker) 1990 The dawn is at hand: selected poems. Jacaranda, Milton

Roberts S L 1978 Behavioural concepts and nursing throughout the life span. Prentice-Hall, Englewood Cliffs

Roy C 1976 Introduction to nursing: an adaptation model. Prentice-Hall, Englewood Cliffs

Sacks O 1984 A leg to stand on. Pan Books (Picador edn), London

Scarry E 1985 The body in pain. Oxford University Press, New York

Scott S, Morgan D (eds) 1993 Body matters: essays in the sociology of the body. Falmer Press, London

Shilling C 1993 The body and social theory. Sage, London

Straus E W and Machado M A 1984 Gabriel Marcel's notion of incarnate being. In: Schlipp P A, Hahn L E (eds) The philosophy of Gabriel Marcel. Open Court Publishing, La Salle, 123–155

Turner B S 1992 Regulating bodies: essays in medical sociology. Routledge, London

Warner S T 1967 T H White: A biography. Cape with Chatto & Windus, London

Woolf V 1967 On being ill. In: Collected essays, Volume 4. Harcourt, New York

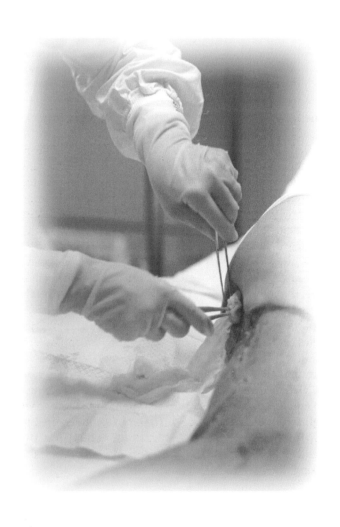

6

Discourses, metaphor and bodies
Boundaries and the skin

Trudy Rudge

Introduction

The notion of embodiment has not, until recently, been a primary focus in our understandings of social action. Further, the dominant perspective in western schemes of knowledge has, from some theoretical perspectives, given pre-eminence to ideas rather than embodiment as a way of understanding human agency and culture (Game 1991). The denial and the taken-for-granted nature of bodies, and their relegation to a secondary position, can be understood as part of the ascendancy of the mind within Enlightenment thinking. A further effect of this has been to focus on theory over and above practice. Much of this can, Leder (1990) suggests, be seen as emerging from the paradoxical nature of embodiment. 'While in one sense the body is the most abiding and inescapable presence in our lives, it is also essentially characterised by absence' (Leder 1990:1). However, it is my contention in this chapter that it is not only the 'lived' experience of our bodies which brings this about. Phenomenological bodily absence is compounded by cultural realities of the ways in which we think and talk about bodies as well as how we act towards our own and others' bodies.

This chapter is an attempt to (re)surface the body's absence in nursing, to analyse and describe the elements that have brought bodies back as a central focus for analysis and to elucidate how these more contemporary approaches afford nursing new insights concerning body care. In so doing, it is hoped to outline the relationship of nursing care to the various bodies and the epistemological and ontological concerns that such new insights emphasise for the discipline of nursing.

Central to this analysis will be much of the contemporary work which suggests that language mediates, shapes and constrains our attempts to understand the place of bodies within our culture and hence within nursing (Cheek & Rudge 1994a). A further concern of the chapter will be to explore how power relations and language use, both metaphoric and discursive, intersect to bring a certain form of body into being and to suggest ways in which this may silence or suppress other possibilities in relation to nurses' thinking and practices towards the body.

The analysis of wound care practices which serve as the basis of this chapter form part of a larger study and as such offer only a partial view of these practices. Moreover, the exploration of how understandings about embodiment intersect with language use in metaphors and discourses will focus on the way skin is represented as 'cover' or 'boundary' in these practices: significant intersections with practices such as class, gender and ethnicity have largely been omitted. While I am aware that without these the picture represented may be too simplistic, the expolorations offered are given in the desire to illuminate the centrality of skin as the emotional, symbolic, socio-cultural *and* physical boundary par excellence (see Anzieu 1989, Grosz 1994).

What is apparent, too, is the way in which these understandings about skin prejudice and influence the way that doctors, nurses and patients talk and think about key aspects of wound care. Metaphors such as obtaining 'cover' and metaphoric explanations used by patients to describe their relationship to both the burnt skin and their 'new' grafted skin, convey certain forms of meaning and frame the practices which surround the experience of burns care. Through analysis of the use of metaphor it is hoped to illuminate the way in which language operates definitionally and to raise some further questions as to how metaphors create possibilities and constraints in the practice setting.

In a similar vein, analysis of discourses evident in wound care practice will further illustrate how language use can no longer be considered as a taken-for-granted background to reality. Rather, language and the meanings it conveys are shown to be neither transparent nor value-free and are permeated with power relations which constitute such meanings. I will focus on further exploration of the ideas and practices around cover, and how these ideas interact with taken-for-granted understandings about independence/dependence. It will be shown that certain forms of body are called forth in these different discursive practices. Crucially, the hope is to convey how language, either as metaphor or discourse, is not independent of bodies but integral to both our thinking and practices towards bodies.

Metaphor as 'embodiments' of meaning?

Recent developments in analyses of nursing practice have turned to considering the centrality of metaphors, and the use of bodily metaphors in particular, as a way of understanding embodiment and nursing practice. Indeed, this is argued as self-evident because nurses, doctors and patients alike frequently use metaphors as a way of communicating the experience of health and illness (see Sontag 1971, Sandelowski 1986, Smith 1992). Moreover, many authors (Jackson 1983, Turner 1984, Johnson 1987) suggest that the body's 'readiness-to-hand', so to speak, may lead to our cultural predilection for bodily metaphors. Johnson (1987) goes so far to suggest that as heuristic devices the importance of bodily metaphors lies as much in our experience of embodiment as in our cultural and historical situations.

Metaphors, as we understand them currently, are ways of explaining one form of reality in terms of another (Fairclough 1989). Central to this point of view is the belief that language is how we represent and interpret this reality (Sarup 1989). Further, until the more recent explorations of metaphor (Turner 1974, Derrida 1976, Lakoff & Johnson 1980 to name but a few), metaphor was considered as a literary device, rather than a form of language use which may be pivotal to both our ability to communicate with others and to understand what is happening in social reality. Indeed, Sarup (1989) emphasises the creative elements of the use of metaphor, in that it can allow us to step outside the bounds of more literal use of language.

Metaphoric thinking imbues not only the everyday reality but also Sarup asserts, following Neitzche, that metaphors are present as explanatory devices in philosophy, science, sociology and the like; and, as Smith (1992) suggests, in nursing theory as well. In particular, Sarup argues that at those points where we are setting out to persuade of the truthfulness of one perspective over another, we are most likely to use figurative language. Importantly, he states that 'attention is now being increasingly given to how rhetorical devices shape our experience and our judgements, how language serves to promote the possibilities of certain kinds of action and exclude the practicability of others' (Sarup 1989:52).

However, as a word of caution to unproblematic acceptance of the primacy of metaphor, Brennan (1993) would suggest that the emphasis on the ubiquity of metaphor is itself driven ideologically. She further asserts that this century's fascination with analyses of metaphor may be a direct result of the need to continue to objectify and distance ourselves from direct experience. Brennan intimates that the very constructedness of our social reality 'might make metaphors more substantial, but they do not make metaphors the only reality, although they may aim to do so' (1993:21). In so doing, Brennan asserts that power is inextricably linked to our use of metaphor.

What I would suggest also is that metaphor has the potential to reinforce hegemonic[1] beliefs and in so doing may act to suppress certain forms of thinking and acting. This occurs from the way that metaphor renders the conditions of experience as if they are common sense. Authors who suggest that metaphor is creative, in that it forges new links, seldom highlight how metaphor can just as well render the world in a taken-for-granted way. Similarly, metaphors may well enhance our predilection for explaining our experience through the use of dichotomies *because* in metaphor we relate one meaning to another. In so doing, we may well be privileging one element of the metaphor and as a result suppressing other potentials offered within the metaphor. Later in this chapter I will return to the question of how this occurs and what the effects on practice may be. Suffice it to say, at this time, that the operations of power are as much in evidence in the form and content of metaphor as in the language form of discourse.

The age of the 'bounded' metaphor

What Brennan is emphasising in her analysis is that certain forms of metaphor continue to dominate even though there are now strong rebuttals against portraying human agency as disembodied and decontextualised (Code 1991, Game 1991). While Leder emphasises such invisibility as issuing from our phenomenological experience of the body, it is apparent also that we find it immeasurably difficult to express, through language, our experience of embodiment. As Brennan suggests, our embodiment remains an unspoken reality precisely because mind/body dualism splits our use of the symbolic realm off from our bodies.

From conceptions of embodiment as our primary ontological focus in understanding our place in society, it is a short step towards theoretical perspectives which view 'the body' as a principal metaphor for interpreting social life. This perspective posits that body metaphors emerge because of the ways we anthropomorphise our 'natural' world to make sense of it (Jackson 1983). Jackson argues that this occurs from the way that metaphors shape our social, cultural and political understandings. Further, metaphor is a productive force, in that it calls into being our world as we experience it (Lakoff & Johnson 1980). It is also a way of conveying meanings which are easily understood *because* it is assumed they are shared. Metaphors of embodiment can therefore be viewed as a primary reference point for either explaining our social situations or social practices as well as a way of explaining our various and infinite relations to our bodies, in both sickness and health.

Sontag (1971), in her now germinal essay *Illness as Metaphor*, outlines the ways in which metaphors of contagion and military struggle inform our understandings concerning cancer; and likewise metaphors concerning cancer inform our social understandings about society such as the cancer of poverty or delinquency. As Turner (1984:113) asserts, 'because the body is the most potent metaphor of society, it is not surprising that disease is the most salient metaphor of structural crisis. All disease is disorder — metaphorically, literally, socially and politically'.

Similarly, Jackson (1983) extends this point by suggesting that while bodily metaphors arising from the experience of health and illness are crucial for understanding some aspects of disorder, personal or social, they also figure strongly in the cultural sphere as a form of thinking and speaking through the body. While it can be argued that such an approach allows an analysis which seeks to explain our predilection for metaphors as solely located *in* our minds, it is critical to remember that this is overlaid by manifold socio-cultural understandings. It is not my intention to convey an essentialist reading of metaphor, neither one that could be interpreted as structural. Rather, as I highlighted in the earlier discussion on metaphor, the meanings that we ascribe to metaphors, especially as they relate to embodiment, are driven by power relations in society (see Brennan 1993). This I contend lies not just in how meaning is conveyed through metaphor, but by the way that metaphor may structure the meaning which is available to us within them. The question still remains as to how metaphor operates hegemonically; how does it co-opt us to support the status quo? In order to offer some suggestions as to how this occurs I will turn to the insights afforded by psychoanalytic theory.

Both Freud and Lacan would suggest that our identities as individuals are first bound to our bodies, through our senses and by the sense of identity provided by skin. Hence Anzieu's (1989) skin ego, which uses Freud's notion of the body ego (Freud 1915). These understandings are expressions of the integrated nature of mind and body; the skin or body representing our physicality and ego as our psychological or mental energies. Anzieu, following Freud and Lacan, views the skin as the organ which provides us with the first understandings of how we are separate ego identities.

This foundational understanding is represented in our psyche by our beliefs that our psyche's energies are as bounded as our skins; that even as we are physically bound by skin, we also are bound psychically. Further, these understandings of how we are separate from each other act at both the conscious and unconscious levels of the psyche. Additionally, and this is a key to understanding how skin conveys our psychic boundaries, our separation at the level of ego through our identity is set socio-culturally through our skin; our skin comes to represent the social and cultural experience of being a self-contained individual. We see ourselves as individuals, bounded and independent one from each other (Lacan 1977, Brennan 1993). As Brennan states,

> ...the social actually gets into the flesh, and unless we take account of this, we cannot account for the extent to which socio-historical realities affect us psychically, and how we in turn act in ways that produce and reinforce them. We also need to address the problem of how we come to experience ourselves as contained entities, contained in terms of energies and affects (1993:10).

It is the containment of both our physical and psychic energy which is hegemonic in character and hence conceived of as natural. When such understandings are mobilised in the metaphors we use to speak about skin, we set up certain possibilities and exclude others from our social, cultural and psychological explanations of our understandings about what skin means to us. Further, metaphors we use to talk about body boundedness act at both the conscious and unconscious level. Following Lacan, I would suggest that the unconscious is mapped with metaphors of boundedness and, as a result, significant parts of their meaning are repressed and hidden from us; just as our conscious energies (practical and theoretical) are largely taken up with continuing to talk and act towards ourselves as if we were unproblematically bounded individuals. It is the notion of the unconscious which assists in conceptualising how our beliefs about boundedness get into our minds (and hearts) with the result that we are co-opted and hence participants in our oppression (Brennan 1993, Weedon 1987).

Further, as Easthope (1986) suggests, following Lacan, this boundedness is best represented in the masculine ideal which he terms 'the citadel of the self'. Brennan (1993) also believes that this notion has currency because of powerful intersections between patriarchy and capitalism, which are meant to deny our connectedness. Indeed, the primacy of bounded metaphors may well have pre-eminence because these metaphors ideologically support these two systems. So not only is the notion of boundedness general, it is more specifically a gendered metaphor, in that the self which is bounded is the masculine self.

I turn now to an exploration of the structuring of thought and action by metaphor which occurs in the care of burns patients to illustrate how metaphors are productive and delimiting of practices. I provide an analysis of what I have come to term 'the will to cover', through exploration of how metaphoric understandings about skin as cover suppress the depth experiences of skin.

Bounded metaphors: the will 'to cover'

One of the central motifs of burns care is that of achieving cover and managing that cover, as well as a variety of 'covering' metaphors used by patients to explain their changed relationship to their burnt or grafted skin. In obtaining cover, the language use conveys understandings about the scientific functions of skin but simultaneously conveys how these practices are as much influenced by the symbolic. It further allows for an understanding of the process of grafting which focuses on the protection offered by 'complete' skin against the onslaughts of the environment — it covers the patient against contagion. As well as this, cover makes invisible again the debrided flesh, completing the boundary between patient and environment which has been ruptured by the burn trauma.

These understandings about skin are both technologically and culturally driven. Cover means closure of boundaries, with all of the symbolic and affective meaning which this entails; as a result, this process motivates much of the care given to burns patients. While many analyses of our relationship to our skin have focused on this boundedness as a way of understanding social practices (Douglas 1966 and 1970) and nursing practices (Lawler 1991), I consider that there is more to this imperative than achieving 'functional' boundaries. In the psychoanalytic theory of Freud and Lacan, and inter-pretations of their work, the centrality of psychic and unconscious forces are exposed for the influence they have on our beliefs about boundedness (Anzieu 1989, Brennan 1993, Grosz 1994). I believe this perspective reveals what is not being spoken about when we focus only on skin as a surface on which we play out our cultural belief systems. To focus on function is to treat skin as if it is a *surface reality*, not something to which we are attached in a rather integral manner.

Moreover, just how integral skin is to our survival is affirmed by how many of the body systems are endangered when only small proportions of the body surface are lost. This physical boundedness is, however, only a part of the story if one is to understand the cultural imperative for cover. In the use of terms such as cover, which putatively have scientific underpinnings, the nurses and doctors are alluding to only the surface functions of skin. They know that skin loss affects more than the surface. However, in the focus on obtaining cover, on how the wound and skin look, on how the grafts look and how effectively they are covering the debrided surface, they are acting towards the skin as if it is *only* surface. As I highlighted previously, notions of boundedness are masculinised, but they are also evocative of the power inhering to masculine scientific thinking. This is so because metaphors which mobilise ideas of humans as being self-contained do not challenge hegemonic beliefs about humans as individuals, complete in and of themselves.

Metaphors of skin as cover not only constitute the contained body but they also, as Brennan (1993) suggests, separate us from each other by the way in which they allow us to distance ourselves, and thus objectify, felt experience. When they talk about wound care, nurses almost invariably point to the visibility of wound healing and the pleasure that this ensures 'when you can actually see the wound healing from day to day'. This form of understanding of wounds and the healing process focuses on the surface of the wound and the skin in almost complete denial of the hidden (psychic) wounds and the hidden aspects of wound healing which occur beyond the visible surface in the depths of the body. In seeking to relate their practice to these surface observations, nurses objectify and reduce the complex interplay of psychological, social and cultural realities of wound care which could allow for some comprehension of the depth experience of skin. Focusing on the visible is to be seduced by the masculinised metaphors of boundedness, in that it views the surface as more controllable than the deeper psychic intensities of skin loss.

In a major study (Rudge, in progress), I have been particularly impressed by the pervasiveness of covering metaphors that is evidenced in the ways that patients talk about being burnt. In attempting to explain how he experienced the effect of full thickness burn to the chest and stomach one patient described that it felt like 'body armour — stiff and not attached to his body underneath'. This same patient said that when he was first grafted, the grafts felt like body armour and equally unattached. Similarly, patients often used technological covering metaphors to convey their understandings about the grafts and dressings used in their care — a curious inversion of metaphor, which in turn conveys much concerning the embodied way in which we comprehend technology (see Haraway 1991). They spoke of the grafted areas as feeling like plastic, or as one older man put it when describing how his new grafts looked — 'like Gladwrap over meat'.[2]

In their struggle to comprehend the new way their skin felt, the patients talked about a novel appreciation of their unaffected skin; they used it as a way of comparing the grafted areas. As one young man put it:

> I mean I touch this bit [grafted section of arm] and I can feel it and it's sort of like you'd think it would be — but then I touch this bit here [touching an unaffected part of his arm] and I know it's different, um, it's sort of tingly, not like skin at all really — like rubber with some sort of sensation. No, it's not like **real skin**.

What seems very evident in the patients' discussion of their burns and grafts, and indeed the way they acted towards them, is the similarity of their approach to that of the doctors and nurses. However, once the graft had taken, and they were starting to move again, what emerges is an understanding of skin as both cover and 'attachment'. What I mean by this is that patients spoke of their skin as covering a depth, integrally attached to them and altering their relationship to the way their body moves. Embedded within this talk is a struggle to re-develop an unproblematic relationship towards their skins.

As both Brennan and Anzieu point out, skin is the location of a double message; both touched and felt. In speaking about how it feels, patients are foregrounding the felt reality of skin from the other side. Moreover, what this also conveys is the way that their skin has been made into other-than-skin because of the trauma. While they talk about the visible aspects of grafts and burnt skin using covering metaphors, they constitute their skin as something which is not self and hence 'other', which can distance them from the experience. On the other hand, they recognise that the skin is theirs — even the donor skin — is 'my skin'. What they struggle to express is the depth experience of the skin, what it feels like from a lived position that nurses and doctors cannot experience. While nurses and doctors talk about grafts looking good, patients talk about what the new skin does to their whole body, and most specifically about being able to move their bodies.

The crucial element highlighted by all of the patients I talked to was how to get their bodies moving again *with* the skin. Further, it is as if there is more to say, but there is little provision made within the dominant covering metaphors for the expression of the patient perspective. While movement is addressed by doctors, nurses and other health workers, this is not about 'the felt' domain of human embodiment but rather about independence: 'the bounded self'. I will now turn to how cover, self care and independence are represented and framed discursively. First I will provide some discussion of discourse as a form of social practice and how discourses can mediate and constitute the body.

Discourse: language as power and knowledge

As with analyses of metaphor, focal issues for such analyses are identification of how language, power, knowledge and various social structures interact to create and reproduce society. As Buchbinder suggests, 'discourse may be thought of as a kind of language about a topic or a preoccupation in the culture' (1994:29). Similarly, for Foucault (1980), discourses were evident in the way thinking and acting were constituted in certain ways by social texts and vice versa. He considered that the process of delimiting social practices, particularly in relation to bodies or the social body, was accomplished by an intimate relationship between power and knowledge and social and institutional practices. Because of this close relation between power and knowledge he came to speak of this relation as power/knowledge. The relation between the use of power and the use of knowledge produced discourses, preoccupations or the currency of certain ideas at particular times.

Further, linking power with the use of language in this way allows us to understand how some ideas and the social practices which they frame may come to seem more 'natural', 'logical' or 'truthful' than others. Central to such scrutiny is the exploration of how one defines 'truth' and makes claims to speak or know the 'truth'. For example, several authors (Foucault 1973, Willis 1994, Cheek & Rudge 1994b) have suggested that the dominance of medical expertise is based on truth claims of medical/scientific discourses and the right this has in turn made available to the medical profession to speak and practise.

There are, however, multiple forms of discourse present at any social moment, all of which are contesting and contestable. It follows from this that there are a multitude of positions available through which one can define, assert and make known the self, as one positions oneself according to the possibilities afforded by certain discourses. For example, within the health care system there is a contest between medical/scientific discourses of medicine and the economic discourses of economic rationalism. This is evident in the debates between medical organisations and the government departments which fund the system whenever various cost-cutting measures are mooted. Doctors, administrators and nurses position themselves in different ways according to these discourses.

Further, the exercise of such power/knowledge is not always employed in a top-down manner, but is in evidence at the very fingertips of society, forming webs of power/knowledge. Such webs of relations structure debates between various discourses over who had the right to speak, who had claims to what knowledge and what position this knowledge would allow the speaker to take in society. Furthermore, it is important to point out that the vision of society which this perspective supports is not what is termed 'a pluralistic society' where all positions are assumed as having equal access to definitional rights (or the idea that power relations may be central is avoided). Instead, as Gavey (1989) suggests, not all discourses are accorded equal definitional ability. Just as discourses reflect dominant positions, and prescribe 'what is said and to whom; and with regard to who is to be "heard" and thus empowered by being given a voice, and who is to be silenced and hence disempowered' (Buchbinder 1994:30), they do allow the possibility of alternative or *resistant* discourses. In so doing, such analyses allow a view of society (and nursing) which avoids the overly deterministic and top-down understandings about power which have a tendency to assume complete suppression of those who resist dominant discourses or frames.

Such a perspective invites analysis of how resistance may lead to alterations in power relations and societal preoccupations over time. Discursive frames, such as those currently offered within medical/scientific discourses in the health care system, do vary in their ability to hold sway over other, resistant, and competing discourses. Thus, in differing sociohistorical periods, discourses change their focus, or lose their powers of persuasion, with corresponding alterations in ways of thinking and acting.

Finally, as with metaphor, discourses are considered to be creative or productive *and* delimiting, and hence producing and reproducing our collective preoccupations, our ways of acting (with our bodies) and ways that we can resist these preoccupations. As Fairclough (1989:17) suggests, discourse is 'language as social practice determined by social structures'.

The care of the self: poststructural analyses of bodies

Of the many authors working in the field of poststructuralism, the work of Foucault has become central in analysis of bodies. Throughout his project, Foucault (1980) focused on the emergence of a variety of the techniques concerning bodies arising from a contest between various discourses. Foucault characterised this process as uncovering a history of the present in the discourses of the past. In his multiple analyses, Foucault developed perspectives on bodies, extending from classical Grecian and Roman discourses on the care of the self (Foucault 1985, 1986), to discourses on sexuality in the 19th and early 20th century (Foucault 1981), as well as discourses that concerned themselves with madness (Foucault 1967), disciplinary practices (Foucault 1977) and medical practices (Foucault 1973). I will not attempt to cover this extensive oeuvre here, but will focus on Foucault's conceptualisation of governmentality, the 'docile body' and his later work on the care of the self, in so far as these are relevant to understanding metaphors of the body in nursing.

Foucault (1977) explains how techniques of surveillance, which he termed panoptic surveillance, reach out from social institutions such as the school, hospital and the prison, to the individual in a manner akin to the capillaries of the body. Such an image of power seeks to overcome the deterministic view of constraint of one group by another, through the exclusive *possession* and exercise of power by a dominant group. Moreover, power is conceived of as a productive force, one that produces the subject, albeit in the form of the docile body. Ultimately, these disciplinary techniques of the body are pervasive, affecting prisoner and prison guard, teacher and student, and doctor and patient equally: an important point for health care workers (Cheek & Rudge 1993).

In his later works on the pleasures and care of the body, Foucault (1981, 1985, 1986, 1988) extends this analysis to the ways in which the body and its care have come to represent the apotheosis of technologies of the individual. These works, on the poststructural concerns of the body, desire, truth claims and the self, concern themselves with techniques of power, domination and resistance. As Foucault (1988:19) presents it, he had come to be 'more and more interested in the interaction between oneself and others and in the technologies of individual domination, the history of how an individual acts upon himself [sic], in the technology of the self'.

In focusing on the issues of sexuality, the articulation of desire and pleasure, as well as the Stoics' care of the self, Foucault (1986) examined these technologies. The aspect of these later works, which is most germane, centres around the notion of self care espoused by the Stoics. Through the processes of self care, the individual was to come to know oneself. By bodily practices or regimens of diet, exercise, the keeping of diaries of reflection and meditation, writing to friends, the individual would come to 'know' himself [sic].[3] Just as

Foucault (1981) finds an urgency for sexual confession in the silencing of sexuality by the Victorians, the Stoics instituted the self as a project to be 'written' into being in diaries and letters to a mentor which chart the course of the exploration into health and purity.

However, Foucault emphasises that these disclosures remained essentially private thoughts about the self. They do not constitute the self as a public entity. Instead, he turns to the rituals of confession instituted by the Christian church, where the individual renounced oneself, one's bodily control and disclosed one's innermost thoughts publicly. The figures of public penitence and martyrdom remain the peculiar preserve of the Christian renunciation of the self. As Foucault (1988:46) states, such self-examination was:

> to examine any thought which presents itself to consciousness to see the relation between act and thought, truth and reality, to see if there is anything in this thought which will move our spirit, provoke our desire, turn our spirit away from God. The scrutiny is based on the idea of a secret concupiscence.

The act of confession that came to dominate in this process of renunciation of the self was verbal self-disclosure, or confession. However, this differs from modern practices of the body and the self in that, in the present, such self-disclosure does not necessarily lead to a renunciation of the self. Instead, self disclosure and work on the self produces a new and transformed self, constituted in and through the act of verbalisation and self-disclosure (Foucault 1988). It is not difficult to recognise that here Foucault is alluding to personal growth groups, motivational seminars and psychoanalytic therapy as confession and transformation, or indeed the setting of personal goals and objectives which obsess educationalists and management theorists alike today. What this also indicates is that there is a politics of surveillance, or governmentality (Foucault 1979, 1988), implicit in such techniques. As with the notion of panoptic surveillance, Foucault is further theorising the intricacies of self-government, and in particular how these processes bring into being the individual as sovereign — a key support to the notion of individual rights in western capitalism.

Integral to explicating such concerns are poststructural perspectives on discourse and the notion of desire (Coward 1984, Weedon 1987, Game 1991, Bordo 1993). Indeed, Game (1991) asserts that in the construction of knowledge about society, one of the sources of our impetus to understand how things work and function is the desire for mastery evident in our search for knowledge and desire to know. However, from the perspectives of all of these authors, such desiring of mastery remains constrained by western philosophy's epistemic focus on objectivity and rationality (Code 1991). All of this intersects with understandings about the self which Foucault alluded to in his later works. It also parallels the notions which I have identified as implicit in the use of metaphors that portray self-containment and masculinised boundedness. Indeed, self-containment is as much in evidence in the desire for mastery of the self and the notion of governmentality which are abundant in discourses surrounding practices of wound care.

85

Politics of wound care, self care and subjectivity

To return to analysis of the politics of wound care, a key discursive framing of nursing centres around notions of self care. Indeed, many nursing theories are predicated, at least partially, on nursing as a process through which the patient re-establishes the ability to self care (Henderson 1969, Nightingale 1969, Orem 1980 to name but a few). There is insufficient space here to trace the history of this discourse, but such is its centrality to nursing that, I believe, it now governs nursing practice, with and for patients, ideologically. Foucault's work on care of the self is germane to this, as is the notion of discourse and ideology.[4] Following Foucault's thesis concerning discourses and the development of governed bodies as subjects of discourse, I contend that discourses on self care constitute certain forms of subjectivities. Indeed, subjectivities, be they nurse, patient or doctor are brought into being as an effect of certain powerful and definitional discourses (Henriques et al 1984, Hollway 1989). Just as Foucault (1979, 1988) explored the discourse of care of the self in relation to government of *and by* the individual, there are apparent within the practices of wound care, discourses which determine how nurses, doctors and patients talk and think about wounds.

Nursing texts are predicated on certain discursively produced understandings of the patient. Indeed, within the rubric of nursing practice, self care is predicated on 'common' understandings concerning the individual, and the effects of illness or disability on an individual. Further, the nursing belief system about independence/dependence also covers aspects about how it is that an individual comes to be independent, moving from one end of the putative continuum to the other. Hence, the goal of much nursing work is to move the patient from the position of dependent patient to that of independent person.

However, in the process of healing following burn trauma this is less of a set pathway, rather in the course of treatment there are movements back and forward between the two poles, returning to high levels of dependency with each return to the operating suite for debridement and skin grafting. Maintenance of a continuing forward movement towards some level of independence is made all the more difficult because of this fluctuating treatment pathway. Given the complexity of this process, how do the discourses of self care operate to shape and form the pathway for patients, nurses and doctors? What form does this contestation take and what are the dominant and resistant frames which form the politics of wound care? Are there similarities, differences or silencing of certain perspectives in evidence in these discourses of self care which operate as ways of talking about wound care?

Wound care, from the perspective which informs this analysis, is a site of intersection of medical technology, cultural understandings concerning the body, and bodily functions in health and illness, as well as the materiality of bodies themselves (see Lupton 1994). As previously outlined a key element of burns care is the achievement of cover: the re-establishment of biological (and subsequent sociopolitical) body boundaries by healing and grafting of debrided areas. Further, there is evidence of competing discourses in the approaches to wound care after burn trauma. I believe that the contest between these discourses is testimony to the illustrative power of practices such as wound care in understanding nursing's relationship to bodies. A primary focus of self care is the taking over of care of the new and healed skin areas by the patient. Underpinning this process are beliefs about the notion of patienthood for doctors, nurses and patients.

As a case in point, a governing frame in burns care is the need to complete the grafting process as quickly as possible, even though in the first few days this may lead to increasing the loss of body boundaries to the point of 'danger', because the donor areas also are then counted as areas of skin loss. This impulse comes from discourses which are evident in medical research as they relate to reduction in death rates from infection due to loss of the skin's function as a boundary against incursion into the body by bacteria — a very necessary concern. This imperative means also that patients return to the operating suite very quickly, about every ten to fourteen days and very quickly after admission — within a few days of admission. This impulse is mentioned not as a point of criticism of the treatment, but as evidence of a dominant constitutive factor for doctors, nurses and patients on this unit. In this sense then, technological discourses interact with notions about self care which lead to a precipitate and rapid progress to cover. At cover, the patient is then considered also to be capable to self care of his/her new skin and the technology which this includes. The doctors seek to make this progress and its components understandable to patients in terms of completing this technological imperative.

At the same time, within the nursing documentation, the variations in self care ability are traced out in the daily reports, in computer generated care plans, and in the observed practice of nurses in the unit. In many ways the nurses resort to the scientific discourses of burn management as constituting the care of the self in the unit. They too, attempt to make understandable to the patient the varying changes to them, the changes in the wound, the different sorts of dressings and their requirements of the patient in the technical process of wound healing. However, this process is not entirely driven by the desire to cover. Nurses seek to find within the daily exigencies of technical care, a foundational sense of the self which arises from making contact with that part of the patient which remains quintessentially, to them at least, independent (May 1992a). With this in mind, notes and plans outline how the patient is to be encouraged to maintain some aspects of self care, even if this is extremely limited by constrained and splinted limbs, limited hand movements and restricted locomotion with lower limb donor sites. Nurses constitute such care as attempts to maintain the patient's notion of themselves.

The desire of many of the nurses was to encourage self care. The discursive framing for such an approach is the belief that if the patient is encouraged to participate in the decision making concerning their care, they have less difficulty in regaining their independence at some future time. However, it is also important to point out that at times while such framing is specific in the notes, nurses in practice allowed patients only some areas of decision making with regard to care. At times considerable effort and space is made for the patient's concerns — at others, all is swept before it in the process of attending to the wound itself. All such actions can use notions of self care prevalent in nursing literature as support for these respective approaches.

The result of such practices is that nurses constitute themselves with regard to the achievement of independence of the patient. Success or failure of the nursing effort (and in some respects other health workers) is measured by how well the patient is able to care for her/himself at the conclusion of their stay in hospital; this is achieved by nurses situating themselves in a 'between' space: between the technology and patient, as interpreter, between the patient and new skin, as primary carer of 'the graft', between the patient and her/his former self, as seeking to encourage independence. As inhabitants of this between space, nurses more frequently call on discourses other than those which are specifically nursing to provide an understanding of the nursing context. They find support for their actions in the scientised discourses of nursing care, as well as those discourses which seek to locate nursing in psychosocial realms (nonscientific in the 'soft' science sense); more recently, nurses are seeing this in the context of the experienced realm and within the concepts of the lived body and embodiment.

But more specifically, as May (1992b) suggests, they incorporate lay understandings as an interpretive bridge for nursing and medical actions in their actions as interpreters of the medical realm. In the ways which nurses act towards ideas such as independence, they are attempting to work in the spaces which remain outside the interest of medical science, and as a point of resistance to the dominant 'covering' frame. When seeking to validate their actions against the scientised norm, the nursing position becomes its most ambiguous and contradictory: when finding its voice within the realm of between, nursing speaks with certitude. However, such understandings about self care, while certain from within nursing discourses, are resisted and contested, not supported as are those which associate themselves with medical-scientific discourses.

From the patients' perspective, the vacillation between independence and dependence is understood more chaotically. Indeed one older patient spoke of it as being on 'a roller coaster ride'. A further impression from this would be that this is a 'ride' over which they had little or no control. They highlight their initial confused state and its continuing effect on their ability to make sense of what is happening. As a counter to this chaos, some patients take on board the scientific and technical aspects of care, searching within the technical knowledge provided by medical and nursing staff for some mastery over the emerging situation. The dominant discursive framing by techniques of wound care, the dressings themselves are an endless source of fascination. Patients can talk about their wound care, the way that the skin looks and know each dressing, its name, what it purports to achieve and what they need to do to care for themselves. It is this aspect of being a patient which finds support from the discursive framings of nurses, doctors and other health workers. What such positioning succeeds in is incorporating the patient into the frame of care of the self as it is defined by medical science and nursing. This is a subjectivity which portrays the patient as becoming independent through expertise; an expert about their 'new' skin and body and in effect the self-governed body.

However, the forming of subjectivity is not such a simple matter. As Weedon (1987) stresses subjectivity is fragmented, contradictory and not entirely authored by the individual. While the attention on self care is centred around patient mastery, this is an understanding not entirely of the patients' authoring: it is framed by the dominant techno-scientific aspects of wound care. As Lawler (1991) suggested of body functioning and nursing practices, such self care is bounded by and given over to the patient, part by part, as the grafting moves to cover. What the patient can rightly care for is defined by the political actions of the expertise of doctors and nurses. Indeed, the reaching of self-mastery is a common understanding by patients, nurses, doctors and other allied health care workers involved in burns care. Such dominant framings bring with them certainty about outcomes and as such provide a commonality, a shared perspective which is completely comprehensible in the light of the need to replace skin and achieve healing through grafting and other forms of wound care.

But there are other aspects of the patients' discursive framing which highlight differences, silencing and resistance to the dominant frames of nursing and medical science. Very many of these concentrate around aspects of understanding about the embodied self which are different. As highlighted earlier, analysis of discursive framing scrutinises how knowledge about bodies, the web of techniques that surround them, allows for 'critiques of the politics of truth' (Smart 1986:166). It is in locating articulations of 'truth', where power/knowledge is most evident. Indeed when such 'truths' are definitional of boundaries within the webs of discourses then the ideas they frame are political; when they are definitional of the boundaries of the body, they are equally political.

Many of the patients report how their bodies felt, how the grafted skin restricted movement and also understood 'the truth' the medical and nursing staff were speaking through direct experience with their 'new' bodies. Patients' discourse differs from that of nurses and doctors, especially as it relates to ideas about independence; elements of patients' subjectivities are silenced and outside this shared and dominant frame of the health professional. Patients talk about their wounds, their relationship to their new body in terms of 'absolute uncertainty'. Their point of reference for 'truth' is not so much in the scientific realities of scar management, but through the 'lens' of the self, at the moment of trauma which in turn has led them to recognise their vulnerability. This uncertainty remains unaffected by information about burn care and scar management. As one patient relates to this 'other' self:

I know that they want me to be more active, but I was always really dependent on [my wife] — I've always looked to her to help me. But on the other hand there is some things that have changed. They will never be the same and this is a chance to change, for the better. I will never do anything so stupid again. I have to think of my wife and kids from now on.

Indeed, nurses', doctors' and health workers' perspectives are future directed towards specific and identifiable aims. Such discourses of independence/dependence are not the same as the uncertainties which the patients share. Regaining such certainty, all of the patients believed, was never going to happen again. In some key way, the burn incident had taken away from them their sense of certainty — over their lives, their bodies and their futures. Indeed one older man even stated that he did not know if this trauma would shorten his life expectancy because of the huge impact he considered the trauma had had on him physically and mentally.

Surrounded as they are by discourses of certainty and 'scientific truths' about the pathway of their illness, such discursive framing of uncertainty is called into being by the frame of the burn trauma itself. It is a deeply resistant, but nevertheless silenced discourse, which is framed by an experience of 'a brush with death'. This is not to deny that many of the patients at the same time became 'the expert' patient in terms of their skin care because subjectivity is intrinsically fragmented and contradictory. While constituting themselves as 'expert patient' gave patients a specific sense of certainty, it did not confront this deep ontological concern with mortality and fallibility which the burn trauma had brought forward. Such understandings about themselves challenge the hegemonic masculinised discourses about self-mastery and independence, as well as the metaphors of self-containment. In some senses the trauma is identified as a crucial element in what most of the patients saw as a transformation. One man said that what he had learnt from being burnt in a bushfire was that he 'was not invincible'. This was further evidenced in ways that patients said that they now had to 'take care', or take each day as it came — a passive, and even feminised response to their forward progress.

While the definition of independence which health workers brought to bear on the attaining of self care was the dominant frame, the patient's framing of the event remained paradoxically at odds with the health workers' more formalised and professional definitional work. The independent self, which the patients saw as irrevocably outside of their present, and potentially their future selves, had been transformed. While gaining more control and a sense of agency with mastery of skin care, there remained a sense of loss of mastery which remained inviolate to scientific truths and to notions of independence. The patients largely saw such independence as unattainable because their relationship to the world had undergone such change that uncertainty was now a permanent way of thinking and acting towards the world; for patients, there were many things which they did not know and were unable to know or predict. The 'citadel of the self' had been penetrated, and much of 'the work' these patients (all men) were now doing was an attempt to come to terms with its continuing repressions and ideological effects from within their changed sensibility.

Conclusion

Poststructural perspectives (re-)open embodiment and theorising about bodies so as to provide fresh insights into epistemic and ontological concerns of nursing and bodies. Such theorising arose from a growing discontent within European philosophy with the Cartesian dichotomy of the mind/body and with the phenomenological accounts of the lived body. Concerning our phenomenological experience of the body, there is indeed an inability to conceive of its presence. Much of the body's work and everyday activities are an unremarkable background to our lives. It is the body's ability to recede from our consciousness to which Leder attributes the power and resonance of the mind/body dichotomy.

However, the consequences of this ontological position are that the body is still viewed as outside dominant masculinised, objective metaphysics. It could also be argued that the approaches of phenomenology fail to come to terms with the processes through which the body comes to be socially defined and constructed by language and structuring social practices. Perspectives which question how and why the body acts as a vehicle of and for cultural reality focus on bodily practices or techniques.

Poststructural perspectives have brought the body back as a central concern for understanding the human condition. The strengths inherent in such an approach also allow the body and the technologies of the body and self to underpin the power and knowledge embedded within certain institutions and core beliefs about individuality. Poststructural analyses also displace the objective reality of the body and replace it with concerns which explore the textual representations of bodies.

Bodies are both object and subject in such discourse, textually mediated realities, an accomplishment of the very discourses which act as the basis of knowledge about bodies. The strengths of these forms of analysis of discursive practices, is that they allow for an interpretation of nursing and nurses' work which seeks to make explicit the politics of nursing care of bodies. Such analyses allow us to recognise the body as the site of contradictions and ambiguities from which no-one is excluded, even those who seek to deconstruct the body and its correlate texts. Moreover, while the dominant frame for much of nursing practice is medical science, nurses and patients alike resist such discursive frames, such resistances opening up a sense of possibilities for other ways of thinking and acting (Cheek & Rudge 1993).

NOTES

1 In using the term hegemonic, I am suggesting that metaphors operate as a way of making the results of dominance appear natural. However, the idea of hegemony, coined by Gramsci (1971), is an important one in that the processes through which hegemony is achieved is that of a constant struggle by the dominant groups to maintain their position. In experiencing the reality of domination, oppressed groups will feel the contradictions of their oppression and hence resist the powers of the dominant groups. Such resistance means that hegemonic beliefs that support the status quo have constantly to be re-won and re-written in order to maintain the power relations which maintain that status quo.

2 Gladwrap is the commercial name of a clear plastic wrapping product. This is an accurate metaphor — the debrided flesh is very visible under the skin when first grafted.

3 This was, as Foucault portrays it, a particularly masculine concern, although Coward (1984) indicates that such concerns are central to the feminine desires represented in the popular culture of women's magazines and in the columns of 'agony aunts'. Many of the 'personal' stories which figure in these forms of media are 'confessional'

in nature, and as a consequence 'surface' female preoccupations and pleasures within the framework of feminine discourses.
4 The notion of ideology which will be used here is underpinned by Foucault's belief that discourse precedes ideology. Ideology can be defined as dominant discursive frames which 'blind' us to other ways of thinking and acting with regard to particular aspects of social life. Such framings are drawn on in taken-for-granted ways which appear 'natural' to us. At the same time as such understandings are employed unproblematically, they also confirm both our specific thoughts and actions and the status quo which they support (see Fairclough 1989).

REFERENCES

Anzieu D 1989 The skin ego. Karnac, London

Bordo S 1993 Unbearable weight: feminism, western culture and the body. University of California Press, Berkeley

Brennan T 1993 History after Lacan. Routledge, London and New York

Buchbinder D 1994 Masculinities and identities. Melbourne University Press, Melbourne

Cheek J, Rudge T 1993 The power of normalisation: Foucauldian perspectives on contemporary Australian health care practices. Australian Journal of Social Issues 28:271–284

Cheek J, Rudge T 1994a Nursing as textually mediated reality. Nursing Inquiry 1:15–22

Cheek J, Rudge T 1994b Webs of documentation. Australian Journal of Communication, 21(2):41–52

Code L 1991 What can she know? feminist theory and the construction of knowledge. Cornell University Press, Ithaca

Coward R 1984 Female desire: women's sexuality today. Paladin, London

Derrida J 1976 Of grammatology. Translated by GS Spivak. Johns Hopkins University Press, Baltimore

Douglas M 1966 Purity and danger. Routledge & Kegan Paul, London

Douglas M 1970 Natural symbols: explorations in cosmology. Barrie & Rockliffe, London

Easthope A 1986 What a man's gotta do: the masculine myth in popular culture. Grafton, London

Fairclough N 1989 Language and power. Longman, London

Foucault M 1967 Madness and civilisation. Tavistock, London

Foucault M 1973 The birth of the clinic: an archaeology of medical perception. Tavistock, London

Foucault M 1977 Discipline and punish. Tavistock, London

Foucault M 1979 Governmentality. Ideology & Consciousness 5 (Summer):5–21

Foucault M 1980 Michel Foucault: power/knowledge: selected interviews & other writings 1972–1977. Gordon C (ed) Pantheon, New York

Foucault M 1981 The history of sexuality, volume I: an introduction. Pelican, Harmondsworth

Foucault M 1985 The use of pleasure. Pantheon, New York

Foucault M 1986 The care of the self. Pantheon, New York

Foucault M 1988 Technologies of the self. In: Martin L H et al (eds) Technologies of the self: a seminar with Michel Foucault. University of Massachusetts Press, Amherst, 16–49.

Freud S 1915 The unconscious. In: Strachey J (ed) Standard Edition, Volume 14. Hogarth, London

Game A 1991 Undoing the social: towards a deconstructive sociology. Open University Press, Milton Keynes

Gavey N 1989 Feminist poststructuralism and discourse analysis: contributions to feminist psychology. Psychology of Women Quarterly, 13:459–475

Gramsci A 1971 Selections from the prison notebooks. Translated and edited by Q Hoare, G Nowell-Smith. Lawrence & Wishart, London

Grosz E 1994 Volatile bodies: towards a corporeal feminism, Allen & Unwin, St Leonards, NSW

Haraway D 1991 Simians, cyborgs and women: the reinvention of nature, Free Association Press, London

Henderson V 1969 Basic principles of nursing care. International Council of Nurses, Geneva

Henriques J, Hollway W, Urwin C, Venn C, Walkerdine V 1984 Changing the subject: psychology, social regulation and subjectivity. Methuen, London

Hollway W 1989 Subjectivity and method in psychology: gender, meaning and science. Sage, London

Jackson M 1983 Thinking through the body: an essay on understanding metaphor. Social Analysis 14(Dec.):127–149

Johnson M 1987 The body in the mind: the bodily basis of meaning and imagination. University of Chicago Press, Chicago

Lacan J 1977 Ecrits: a selection. Translated by A Sheridan. Tavistock, London

Lakoff G, Johnson, M 1980 Metaphors we live by. University of Chicago Press, Chicago

Lawler J 1991 Behind the screens: nursing, somology, and the problem of the body. Churchill Livingstone, Melbourne

Leder D 1990 The absent body. University of Chicago Press, Chicago

Lupton D 1994 Medicine as culture: illness, disease and the body in Western societies. Sage, London

May C 1992a Nursing work, nurse's knowledge, and the subjectification of the patient. Sociology of Health and Illness 13(4):472–487

May C 1992b Individual care? power and subjectivity in therapeutic relationships. Sociology, 26(4):589–602

Nightingale F 1969 Notes on nursing: what it is and what it is not. Dover, New York

Orem D E 1980 Nursing: concepts of practice, 2nd edn. McGraw Hill, New York

Sandelowski M 1986 Sophie's choice: a metaphor for infertility. Health Care for Women International 7:439–453

Sarup M 1989 An introductory guide to post-structuralism and postmodernism. University of Georgia Press, Athens, GA

Smart B 1986 The politics of truth and the problem of hegemony. In: Hoy D (ed) Foucault: a critical reader. Basil Blackwell, Oxford, 157–173

Smith M 1992 Metaphor in nursing theory. Nursing Science Quarterly 5(2):48–49

Sontag S 1971 Illness as metaphor. Farrar, Straus and Giroux, New York

Turner B S 1984 The body and society: exploration in social theory. Basil Blackwell, Oxford

Turner V 1974 Dramas, fields, and metaphors: symbolic action in human society. Cornell University Press, Ithaca and London

Weedon C 1987 Feminist practice and poststructuralist theory. Basil Blackwell, Oxford

Willis E 1994 Illness and social relations: issues in the sociology of health care. Allen & Unwin, Sydney

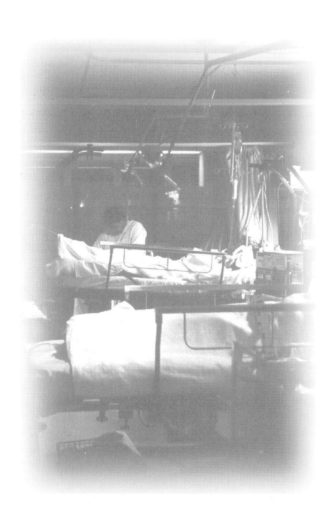

7

The body, the person, technologies and nursing

Pamela van der Riet

Introduction

The issues that are the focus of attention in this chapter centre on the relationships between technologically oriented care, nursing practice and the human body. I will explore the close relationship between technology (including technological support and intervention), nursing care, medical practice(s), the medical model and notions of caring for the person-in-the-body (cf. Lawler, this volume) as well as the physical body. I will be drawing on cases from my own clinical work which reflect the bridge between philosophy, theory and the real world of nursing practice.

The body and the political context of medical care

What is this thing called the body? There are many views. According to Foucault (1981:103–104, 152), the body should not and cannot be just a biological entity; it is a body which is inscribed by history and endowed with power and domination. To Dickson (1990:25) our bodies are 'places where societal practices and organisations of power meet'. Kanner (1993:163) writes that the body is 'represented-constructed, inscribed, attached, described by the cultural systems in which it has physical residence'; and subsequently, the body has become 'a metaphorical custodian of knowledge and power'.

In phenomenological and existential terms, the experience of being human is fundamentally an embodied one. In Sartre's view (cited in Turner 1984:52), one's lived experience in the world is always from one's point of view of one's own body. Phenomenologists argue that people have direct control over their bodies (Turner 1984:57). While this may be true in 'ordinary' daily life, it is an assumption that may not hold up in circumstances of illness and sudden physical distress. In the contexts of health care, the body is regulated by discourses such as medicine and nursing; and patients, who are experiencing the world and their bodies in often unfamiliar ways, do not necessarily have control over their own bodies. Furthermore, their bodies are exposed to inspection and surveillance over which they can have little influence (Turner 1984:58).

Patients are coerced or encouraged and expected to confess their inner secrets to doctors and nurses and other health professionals. They are often dis-empowered by their circumstances and, in many instances, are unaware of their rights to protect themselves and their privacy. The nursing history is testimony to patients being expected to conform to levels of personal exposure — all for the sake of a 'good' medical or comprehensive history, which, allegedly enables health professionals to feel as though they are giving 'good professional care'!

Turner (1884:34) also asserts that the body is a product of political/power relationships; it is an 'object of power produced in order to be controlled, identified and reproduced'. The medicalisation of the body is an example of control and power exerted by the medical discourse. The body is invested with power and it is through the use of language that the body becomes the location where social practices and power meet (Doering 1992:25). Armstrong (1983:41) observed also that 'for Foucault the concept of the body which emerged at the end of the eighteenth century — discrete, objective, passive, analysable — was the effect as well as the object of the medical inquiry'.

Power has both negative and positive attributes; in its negative sense, power excludes, represses, censors, abstracts, masks and conceals (Armstrong 1983:117). Foucault's work established the body as a site at which that power was exercised, indeed, Armstrong (1983:2) suggests that Foucault viewed the body in medicine as political anatomy. It is political because the changes in the way the body is described are based on power which pervades the body.

However, in its positive sense, 'power produces; it produces reality; it produces domains of objects and rituals of truth' (Foucault cited in Armstrong 1983:117). One might question whose notions of truth and power are being discussed or privileged in this setting.

Medical discourses as regimes of body power

Medical discourse, like other dominant discourses, operates as an institution of social control (Willis 1994:6). Whether this control is benign or repressive depends on the discourse in which you are operating. Nursing for example, both in relation to its practice and the articulation of its knowledge, has been repressed by medical discourse. (This is the argument that Lawler explores in chapter two of this volume.)

Scott and Morgan (1993:16) write that 'bodies within organisational hierarchies are controlled and disciplined, their movements clearly defined in terms of time and space'. Clearly in hospital the patient's body is controlled and disciplined. Patients can be subjected to rules that govern when they can have visitors, when to eat, drink, shower and eliminate body wastes. From the time the person enters and leaves hospital they are at risk of being stripped of their own clothing, their body tagged with an identifying (signifying) arm or leg band — their identity is re-framed in reference to their ailments, diagnoses, treatment, or investigations. In effect, their identities become inscribed with medicalised meanings.

Guillaumin (1993:42) argues that surgery (whether professional performed or not), in modifying the body, effects a corporal transformation. He cites, as an example, how sexual mutilation 'surgery', which is permanent, depicts social control over the physical body; and through that physical control, the person is consequentially controlled or constrained. Plastic surgery is another example of transformation, ideally resulting in 'the beautiful body'. However, if the surgery goes horribly wrong it may mutilate and transform the body into an ugly one. Case(s) of breast implantation surgery are the most often cited examples in which the outcome may be a disfigured physical body and a disabled and distressed person. Bordo argues that '[t]he dark underside of the practices of body transformation and re-arrangement reveals botched and sometimes fatal operations' (1991:110).

Technology has provided the tools and the social environment for modifying the body; and various techniques and technologies, both material and experienced, can be harnessed for physical and embodied transformation. In transforming parts of the body one is able to exert control over one's sense of the embodied person. Those who are most vulnerable to the technologies of health care are the ones who have been traditionally powerless. Conversely, those who are most able to harness the technologies of health care for their own ends are the most powerful and privileged. I would argue that women in particular fall into both of these categories — the former more so than the latter. Which is not to say that men are not also vulnerable. However, historically women's bodies have always been targeted, technologised, pathologised and medicalised much more so than have men's bodies

Technologies of medicine and health care

Willis (1994:19) argues for a definition of technology that includes both a material component (machines and tools) and a social component such that 'the development of technology is seen as a consequence of the general process of industrialism, which all modern societies are undergoing'. To Willis (1994:36), social relations are important because they are the means by which patterns of control are dictated within the health system; furthermore, they determine the choice of particular technologies. This is about power and control. What is not always obvious or explicit is the extent to which new technologies in medicine can actually dictate social relations.

Cassell (1991:22) reminds us that in intensive care, which typically is highly technologised, all eyes go to the machinery, rather than to the patient. This is, in part, the seductive power of technology. He argues that it requires effort not to watch the monitors [because] technology — machines, instruments, drug treatment — like blinkers on a horse, restrict and define and thus simplify the viewpoint...[however] unlike blinkers, technology also defines the values that represent good or bad, success or failure. The values of technology are unambiguous and non metaphysical, unlike the other things in the clinical world (Cassell 1991:22).

Technology, machines and tools and access to services are becoming over-riding themes in treatment and diagnosis in medicine — a situation that is leading to further disembodiment (or depersonalising) of people. The body, like technology, is viewed as a machine: it is able to be controlled and manipulated. However, the person inside the body is not a machine, and left with a sense of alienation, might ask 'does this body still belong to me?' Recently I talked with a woman whose brother had been diagnosed with chronic renal failure. She described the difficulty her brother was experiencing with haemodialysis; his body had become 'other' and seeing his blood in tubes outside his body was abhorrent to him. In the process of his body being technologised for dialysis, his sense of personhood and selfhood had become stripped of it familiar identity. The context of this experience had defined his reality into one of disembodiment and rupture. Interestingly, he could tolerate peritoneal dialysis, but not haemodialysis. Subsequently, and despite considerable pressure from his doctors to undertake haemodialysis, he chose peritoneal dialysis because it felt less disruptive and invasive to him as a person.

Both technology and hierarchy have a dialectic effect, that is, they both influence each other (Willis 1994:36) and this is starkly apparent in health care — a major institution of the state. The state in turn has granted and supported 'the dominance of doctors on the division of labour' (Willis 1994:38). Many would argue that this situation results from the knowledge that medical practitioners possess (Illich cited in Willis 1994:38). However, while much of their knowledge/power is illusionary, they are frequently the gatekeepers to our research and knowledge generation, particularly in relation to formalised and public processes through which knowledge about health and illness is acquired, refined and used. In recent years, this tension has been especially apparent when nurses have attempted to conduct research in clinical settings where doctors' power is often overtly exercised.

In seeking ethics approvals from hospitals to conduct research, nurses often encounter the proviso that approval to conduct the research is contingent upon getting the attending doctor's approval to approach 'their patients' for inclusion in nursing projects. In many instances this approval has been denied; in many of these cases the potential research participants are never aware that such decisions, which affect them, have been made. As I have pointed out elsewhere (van der Riet 1993c), the question, among others, that needs to be asked is: who owns the patient's body?

Medical technology, in the quest for 'advancing' health care, must apparently always be the latest and most powerful weapon against disease. New and often more expensive technologies are constantly replacing the old, and technical skill has to be constantly renewed (Willis, Daly & McDonald 1994:86). Like other male dominated fields that rely on machines to help them achieve their goals (such as the military), the medical profession is constantly in search of the latest 'toys' and technical support. Increasing reliance on these technologies (toys) allows unprecedented access to people's physical bodies. The danger here lies in rendering the personhood of the patient more redundant or marginal; the technical equipment is inevitably directed at investigating, supporting and interfering with biophysical phenomena and not lived experiences. Consequently, the body has become involved as a metaphor for the playground in a game with the latest toy(s). There is a site of play with(in) the body. Many times, whilst working in intensive care, I have seen a patient's body surrounded by a virtual sea of equipment and subjected to an obscene display in which health professionals have explored the wonders of their new toy(s), oblivious to the experience of or effects upon the frightened person inside the body.

These technologies are, I suspect, also rendering redundant the ability to care, at least in the sense that we understand this term as meaning something intrinsic as human-to-human interpersonal contact. In many ways, to view technologised medical practices as 'care' is inappropriate and incompatible because with much technologised 'care' and treatment the body is objectified and stripped of the qualities that construct personhood — the person is not being cared for, rather a disease is being investigated and/or treated.

Parker (1992:71) says that

> the body is experienced in a complex way. It is both a centre of one's experiencing but it is also a monitor by which one judges and assesses one's experiences [and that it] becomes an object of interest or concern, while at the same time it remains the centre of one's experiencing.

She argues further that medical discourse develops and relies upon a technocratic imperative which involves the belief that if the technology is available everything technically possible should be utilised to cure and control and thus prevent death (Parker 1992:45). In medical discourse 'cure' or diagnosis are central concerns, whereas in nursing, central concerns are not as fixed on the physical body as an object that contains secrets to be understood and investigated.

Technology, nursing and the body: reflections on technology and care

When nursing is positioned within the 'hard' science paradigm, on which medicine is partly reliant, object is privileged over subject; and this is reflected in the language and practice(s) of modern health care. Bakhtin (1990:288–289) believes that 'language is like the living concrete environment and is never unitary' and that language embraces specific content, judgements and values that knit together and result in particular types of expressions used by the professions.

The language of scientised, medicalised and technologised practices renders the person as object, which poses a dilemma for students of nursing struggling to understand the complexity of nursing. This dilemma is captured in the following student's comments. The student had been working in Accident and Emergency (A & E) and had admitted a sixty-seven year old patient who had been flying a glider plane. The patient had developed chest pain, landed the plane safely and then had a cardiac arrest. In resuscitating the patient the student became caught up in the excitement and adrenalin rush. There was evidence that she had taken up the discourse and professional demeanour of treating the patient as an object.

However, after the initial excitement subsided, she switched to treating the patient as a subject. Her experience is summarised in her reflective case study:

> He looked vulnerable and alone. In this sea of technology a human body looked out of place.
>
> I tried to imagine that this body had a life with his family and flying gliders. I wondered what it would be like to know this person and what he would have to say to us if he were conscious. I found myself (mentally) telling him that he had a massive heart attack and there was not much more our technology and skills could do. A lot of it was up to him. I didn't want to think that he might not make it — he might hear me. This communication occurred inside my mind, where I didn't feel silly for talking to someone who couldn't hear me or respond. None of the nurses or doctors talked to him or acknowledged that he was a human being in any personal way, though they did what they could for his dying body.
>
> I didn't feel like I could touch him, he was cold and bluish like a cadaver. It was still difficult to think of him as human and the one instance when a nurse did talk to him she seemed to do it for my benefit and not his. She looked at me before she catheterised Mr D and I suspect the thoughts about Mr D's dehumanisation were displayed on my face. Before she injected the xylocaine into his penis she told him 'this will be bit cold'. I thought more explanation was needed for such a procedure. But neither did I say anything or explain. Next time, I will try to overcome my fears of appearing foolish or will challenge the actions of the medical and nursing staff.

Technology and technologised environments have the potential effect of disconnecting the person from the body, particularly in environments where the whole ambience is constructed around the technology. I will be drawing on some of my own experiences to illustrate this point.

In ICU for example, I can find myself so involved with the equipment that I forget about connecting with the patient. In a sense I hate this but I am anxious that the patient is cared for 'properly', that is, that all of the technical aids are used to support the patient and their care. Ironically though, the equipment prevents the patient being cared for (in what I perceive to be a caring manner) because I am not connecting with the patient as a living person but instead with the equipment and through it (indirectly) to the patient and what it is doing for, or to, their living physical body.

Nurses regularly work with paradoxes such as this. For example, several years ago I was nursing a patient with congestive cardiac failure in an intensive care unit; he was dying and had been assigned the infamous 'not for resuscitation' tag (van der Riet 1994:95). He was, however, on a dopamine infusion, which was ineffective in his case, and after I had notified his wife at 5 a.m. of his deterioration, the doctor increased his dopamine infusion to the maximum rate. This meant that I had to change the patient's infusion line and work out the rate for this altered dose. Consequently, I had to spend time tending to technology for debatable and dubious purposes when I could have spent time with the patient and his wife.

I felt frustrated and angry over this incident yet it seemed to heighten my awareness of how easily the medical/technical domain became the immediate priority, rather than a more human-oriented approach that could privilege comfort and dignity; that is, I faced the dilemma of technologies and the power of medicine versus my concern for the person. This was all time wasted, in my view, because I had to attend to the machinery instead of spending time with the dying patient and his wife and seeing them as people. I felt frustrated and angry over this incident. The intrusion of the technically privileged approach to this dying man's care seemed so inappropriate because only a few hours earlier the patient had requested that I stay with him. I had done this, and also spent time gently stroking his face, arms and hands until he lapsed into a coma.

According to Foucault (1991:138), hospitals are like prisons, schools and factories, in that they all produce the docile body. This docile body, in westernised health care practice, is subjected to technologically oriented treatment which frequently renders the body powerless in the face of machinery and equipment, just as the person can be powerless in an experienced, social sense. It is also the case that the technology (equipment) itself both demands and produces docility.

In the Cartesianism that is characteristic of scientised discourses and practice, there exists a mind/body schism in the way much health care is delivered, administered, and experienced. In health care, this schism is exacerbated through ever-increasing means of extending the panopticism and clinical gaze that Foucault (1976, 1991) articulated; advances in technology now permit a much more penetrating, in-depth gaze of the physical body (Cassell 1991:174). This gaze is extended beyond the surfaces of whole bodies to the deeper and more mysterious hidden parts of the internal body, which is often transformed in three dimensional, living (and sometimes) moving colour as it is investigated for sources and locations for pathology. There is an ever increasing capacity to examine our own innards and to have them open (so to speak) to a relatively public gaze and to have a growing number of our biological processes monitored, often in extraordinary detail, and manipulated (that is, treated).

Illness, as an experienced phenomenon, is not a single event but a process which is essentially social rather than biological (Willis, Daly & McDonald 1994:99). However, 'the relationships through which...technology is applied constitute the patients as "objects", whereas those in which...patients are more actively involved help to form them as "subjects" ' (Willis et al 1994:99).

Further to this, Willis et al (1994:99) argue that when patients act as subjects, their medical practitioners also become engaged as subjects, yet medical discourse is the medium and the means through which the patient is positioned as subject or object. Generally, the patient is positioned as object. Essentially, what I am arguing here is that this is about power and position; about medical power that positions the patients as objects. Nurses also collude in this by the language that they use and the positions they adopt vis-a-vis the patient. They can position themselves with power *over* the patient rather than *with* the patient. The former results in distancing and a lack of acknowledgment of the person's selfhood, is non-caring and non-therapeutic.

In our highly technologised world of practise on and with the body of the patient, one needs to raise the question: what now? What are the theoretical/ philosophical and practical problems and implications for nursing?

There are issues of privacy, suffering, dignity, intimacy, ethics, spirituality and caring which are often ignored, marginalised, or acknowledged as an afterthought. Often, the patient's lived experience of illness (subjectivity) is disregarded. The person-in-the body is lost and forgotten (one might even say abandoned), yet their pathology receives overwhelming attention and discussion!

Technology, the technical environment and nursing practice

In a major study of the use of complementary therapies in nursing education I was able to examine some of the salient aspects that differentiate technical and more personal(ised) nursing care (van der Riet 1993a). I will be drawing from this study to illustrate that technology and more embodied-subjective approaches to nursing practice are not always compatible and that fractures between the two are apparent in both discourse and practice.

There are also aspects of nursing care where distinctions cannot be made in a dichotomous way because they are complex acts; in other circumstances, it is possible to provide physical care in a technically competent way without any investment from the person of the nurse. In other situations and for other acts, it is not for the nurse to simply perform technical acts without a personal investment in what is being done. For instance, the giving of a pethidine injection can be both an impersonal and technical act, or it can be almost totally technical in the way it is performed. In contrast, a massage cannot be successful if it is conducted as a purely technical performance.

The students I studied as they learned to use massage in their practice set up dualisms in their talk — making distinctions between the technical aspects of practice and the other, that is the alternative.

Tania:	*You almost feel as though you have achieved more* [by giving the patient a massage], *better than giving them a pethidine injection*
Katrina:	*Yeah* (A discussion with the others ensues. They nod their heads in agreement)
Katrina:	*It opens up — they* [patients] *talk to you more*
Other Students:	*Yeah*
P vdR:	*So what is it about the massage? What does it seem to facilitate?*
Katrina:	*I think it shows that you are caring about them*

The discursive field of nursing is informed by both science and the arts, however, there is a tension here between the two. Lawler (1991a, 1991b) addresses this tension and argues for a somological approach to nursing practice, which integrates both what is objectively real, but also includes the subjectivity of the patient such as the lived body experience. She argues for a balanced perspective by viewing those aspects of nursing that have been traditionally framed as both nursing-as-art and nursing-as-science though she rejects the science-versus-art debate as a possible position (1991a, 1991b). My argument is that if nursing makes claims to be more scientific than artistic it may be at risk of losing the ethic of caring.

Caring in nursing is problematic because the system does not value nor support caring (Morse et al 1990:3-4). Even though caring in its various meanings is central to nursing, the hospital environment often precludes caring or severely restricts it. For example, hospitals are frequently understaffed and the increased demand of technology for technological skills often conflicts with nurses' ability to practise in the way they would like.

The intensive care environment, for example, is often tense and noisy. Privacy is frequently non-existent. Acutely ill patients are subjected to round-the-clock treatment. Subsequently, patients can experience sensory overload as every orifice is invaded by some technical apparatus. This all adds to a sense of lost personhood as the body forms a seamless blend with the technical environment and individual pieces of equipment; the body becomes technologised and objectified.

Recently, whilst I was supervising students on their clinical practicum, a second-year nursing student spoke to me about her distress over an experience in the day surgery theatre. She had just observed a patient undergoing electro convulsive therapy (ECT) for depression. What she found most distressing was the way the patient was treated as an object without any sense of respect for personhood. For example, she heard the doctor say at the completion of the procedure, 'Well, that was great, we were able to get 100 more volts into him this week!' She observed that, 'It was as if his body was a mere piece of meat!'

Martin (1989:19–20) has addressed this issue, arguing that

> many elements of modern and medical science have been held to contribute to a fragmentation of the unity of the person [because] when science treats the person as a machine and assumes the body can be fixed by mechanical manipulations, it ignores and it encourages us to ignore, other aspects of our selves, such as our emotions or our relations with other people.

103

There is a growing literature showing that patients in intensive care environments have felt the intrusion of equipment to be anxiety producing and alienating (Fitter 1986), and that technology and technological acts contribute to depersonalised care because they are barriers to touching (Sinclair 1988). On many occasions while working in intensive care I have reminded friends and relatives that it is okay to touch the patient; their response has usually been one of surprise at being permitted to do something that, in other contexts, would be taken for granted.

The (re)emergence of complementary therapies and massage in nursing practice

It is my argument that massage, which acknowledges the embodied and experiential elements of human life, rejects the technological approach characteristic of technologised medical practice and discourse. In the last decade in particular, many nurses have moved out of this medical/technological discourse into a discourse of the embodied other, partaking through their return to massage (and other therapies) as a part of a repertoire of nursing acts that do not rely on sophisticated technology.

In an institution such as the hospital environment, nursing often means slipping in and out of the two discourses — modern medicine and traditional nursing practice. Often it means that the nurse must daily find a way of juggling the competing demands of technologised care — as the medical practitioners would have it visited upon 'their' patients, and the nurse's own views about what course of action is the most humane and appropriate in a given set of circumstances. Some nurses find a way of managing this balancing act, some find themselves more comfortable in the discourses and practices of modern medicine; however, many opt out, choosing instead to work in less westernised paradigms of what health and illness represent.

Some nurses have rejected (almost totally) the technological discourse. They have become independent practitioners setting up their own massage practice (Brown 1991, Crutch 1991). According to the literature, a number of nurses have left hospital institutions because of dissatisfaction with the medical and technical discourse (Harper 1990, Landon 1990, Orrock 1990, Brown 1991, Crutch 1991) and the power of the dominant discourse to determine care. Increasingly, nurses are becoming disenchanted with the growing influence of economic discourses, which have the potential to, at least partially, supplant or challenge medical power and medicalised discourses.

Gates argues that 'there is a general rejection of purely orthodox medicine because it has become technological and specialised, with little emphasis on fundamental healing' (1994:44). The move from orthodox medical practices to so-called 'complementary therapies' reflects this rejection of technological discourse and the practices that disembody, depersonalise and dehumanise 'care'. I use the word 'care' here advisedly because it is becoming more difficult to describe some medical practices as 'care'.

104

Sims (1986:50) argues that massage, in particular, is a way to counteract the negative effects of illness and hospitalisation because it has the potential to counteract the stress of illness and hospitalisation. This view is supported by my research, which showed that massage was one way to counteract the dehumanising effects of hospitalisation (van der Riet 1993a:43).

Complementary therapies, however, have been criticised within medical discourses because they are perceived to be unscientific (Willis 1994:65); yet they are self-evidently and often purposefully so. The underlying 'truth' behind such criticisms is the unquestioned efficacy and adequacy of science to provide explanations about events in health care. An example from my own career demonstrates this point well. Two years ago a medical practitioner wrote to the editor of a multi-disciplinary journal in which an article of mine 'Effect of Therapeutic Massage on pre-operative anxiety in a rural hospital' had been published (van der Riet 1993b, 1993c). His letter, in part, read as follows:

> The article, 'Effect of Therapeutic Massage on pre-operative anxiety in a rural hospital', contains the phrase 'reflexology is a form of massage involving pressure points on the feet and hands which correlates with specific parts of the body.'
>
> There is no scientific evidence at all to validate the latter part of the statement. The fact that the author uses this method of massage and implies its effect through the above mechanism calls into serious question the scientific competence and your journal's integrity for accepting this statement at face value. It may well be that massage has a (possible?) (favourable?) effect on patients' pre-operative anxieties, but this should be established scientifically, not with any reference to nonsensical practices such as reflexology which has no scientific basis whatever, and with a much larger group of patients.

I responded to his letter pointing out that '...reflexology has been around for thousands of years and historically an established practice of the Ancient Egyptians... ' and explaining various elements of the research design and methodology that would meet accepted standards of scientific rigour.

This medical practitioner's views, sadly, reflect the intellectual arrogance embedded in the view that a biomedical model of medicine is the only legitimate one. I was puzzled why he has attempted to discredit this whole study as unscientific, particularly when, methodologically, it conformed to established scientific methodology. However, the editorial board of the journal decided eventually that it would not be politically correct to publish either of the letters; as a result, the debate which could have heightened awareness and focused attention on an expanding area of nursing was held back. In many ways, this is another example of how the technology of power is exercised through gatekeeping; as a consequence, the dominant ideologies and paradigms of knowledge went uncontested. Likewise, my research was not given the opportunity to be debated in the public domain.

What gets lost in this type of argument is the possibility of alternative ways of understanding how embodied humans respond to a vast array of events and experiences. What also gets lost is the sometimes serious tension associated with establishing the efficacy of complementary therapies using the established benchmarks of traditional scientific rigour. It has been said that the term, 'alternative' is counterproductive in the sense that it does not reflect the present move towards convergence of the different paradigms of health knowledge (Willis 1994:65–72). Increasingly, evidence is coming forward to show that people explore a range of ways to make sense of and manage their illnesses and diseases.

Conclusion

This chapter addresses some of the tensions between the relationship of technology, nursing and the body. The positivistic medical discourse is very strong in nursing and is influenced by technology. The discourse of power has been highlighted and is linked with knowledge which underpins the technological discourse. As Willis points out: 'we need to consider the way that technology interacts with society, rather than how technology determines societal response' (1994:24).

Throughout this chapter the tension between the subject and the object body is also felt. It is argued that the body needs to become a subject of care rather than an object of care. Frequently technology results in the body becoming an object which has been stripped of personhood and disembodied. Whilst we need to have a technical discourse, we need to ensure that it does not become the hegemonic one whereby the body continuously becomes the object and pathologised body.

REFERENCES

Armstrong D 1983 Political anatomy of the body. Cambridge, Melbourne
Bakhtin M 1990 The dialogic imagination. Four essays. University of Texas Press, Austin
Bordo S 1991 'Material girl'. The effacements of postmodern culture. In: Goldstein L (ed) The female body. University of Michigan Press
Cassell E 1991 The nature of suffering. Oxford University Press, Oxford
Dickson G 1990 A feminist poststructuralist analysis of the knowledge of menopause. Advances in Nursing Science 12(3):15–31
Doering L 1992 Power and knowledge in nursing: a feminist poststructuralist view. Advances in Nursing Science 14(4):4–33
Ehrenreich J 1993 Reading the social body. University of Iowa Press, Iowa City
Fitter M 1986 The impact of technology on workers and patients in the health services: (physical and psychological stress). Office for official Publications of the European Communities, Luxembourg
Foucault M 1976 The birth of the clinic. Tavistock, London
Foucault M 1981 The history of sexuality, volume 1: an introduction. Penguin, Middlesex
Foucault M 1991 Discipline and punish. The birth of the prison. Penguin, London
Gates B 1994 The use of complementary and alternative therapies in health care: a selected review of the literature and discussion of the implications for nurse practitioners and health care managers. Journal of Clinical Nursing 3:43–47

Guillaumin 1993 The constructed body. In: Burroughs C, Ehrenreich J (eds) Reading the social body. University of Iowa Press, Iowa City

Harper W 1990 A new world of change. The Lamp 47(4):23

Kanner M 1993 Drinking themselves to life, or the body in the bottle. In: Burroughs C, Ehrenreich J (eds) Reading the social body. University of Iowa Press, Iowa City

Landon P 1990 Caring in the centre. The Lamp, 47(4):24

Lawler J 1991a Behind the screens: nursing, somology, and the problem of the body. Churchill Livingstone, Melbourne

Lawler J 1991b What you see is not always what you get; seeing, feeling and researching nursing. In: Nursing research: Pro-active vs Reactive, Centre for Nursing Research Inc & Royal College of Nursing, Australia, Adelaide

Martin E 1989 The women in the body. Open University Press, Milton Keynes

Morse J, Solberg S, Neander W, Bottorff J, Johnson J 1990 Concepts of caring and caring as a concept. Advances in Nursing Science 1 (1):1–14

Orrock P 1990 Natural therapies - a nursing perspective. The primary care practitioner. The Lamp, (5):21–22

Parker J 1992 Cancer passage: continuity and discontinuity In terminal illness. A study of ways of being in the world with cancer. Monographic Series. Royal College of Nursing, Australia

Scott S, Morgan D (ed) 1993 Body matters. Falmer Press, London

Sims S 1986 Occasional paper. Slow stroke massage for cancer patients. Nursing Times 82(13):47–50

Sinclair V 1988 High technology in critical care: implications for nursing's role and practice. Focus on Critical Care, 15(4):36–41

Smith S 1993 Subjectivity, identity and the body. Indiana University Press, Bloomington

Turner B 1984 The body and society. Basil Blackwell, Oxford

van der Riet P 1993a Complementary therapies in nursing Education. MEd dissertation. University of New England

van der Riet P 1993b Effects of therapeutic massage on pre-operative anxiety in a rural hospital, Part one. The Australian Journal of Rural Health, 1(4):11–16

van der Riet P 1993c Effects of therapeutic massage on pre-operative anxiety in a rural hospital, Part two. The Australian Journal of Rural Health, 1(4):17–16

van der Riet, P 1994 A night shift in ICU. Contemporary Nurse 3(2):95–96

Willis E 1994 Illness and social relations. Allen & Unwin, St Leonards

Willis E, Daly J, McDonald I 1994 The social relations of medical technology: the case of echocardiography. In: Willis E (ed) Illness and social relations. Allen & Unwin, St Leonards

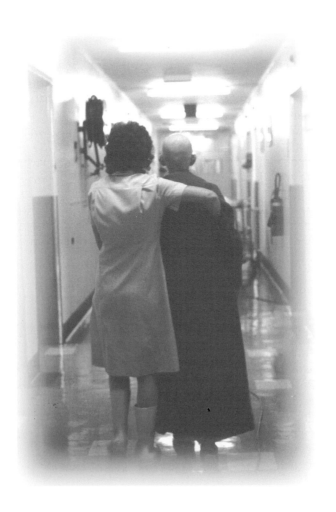

8

The feminised body in illness

Judy Lumby

Introduction

This chapter aims to question the natural scientific assumptions which shape the particular way in which medical theory and practice genders the body, that is, the traditional presupposition that gender attributions 'are natural categories for which biological explanations are appropriate and even necessary' (Bleier cited in Laqueur 1992). Because women's bodies have been readily reduced to their reproductive activities, this chapter will primarily address the female body. The experiences of women living with a life-threatening illness will be used to illustrate some of the problems inherent in the process of essentialising gender categories. Alternative positions will then be posed with a view to suggesting more appropriate models for addressing the fundamental concern of nursing practice: the 'lived' experience of the patient.

Without reducing all science or medicine to one theoretical position or even similar positions, it is possible to identify assumptions, beliefs and processes aligned to scientific thought that inform traditional medical practice. These assumptions include a belief in being able to produce propositions about the natural world through empirical inquiry and reductionist methods. The beliefs and assumptions inherent in scientific approaches to health have had an impact in the way in which health care has been structured and practised. The emphasis has been on institutional care, technological interventions and categorisation of disease premised on an organic way of understanding. Such presuppositions have impacted profoundly on 'sick' individuals in society who consult the doctor expecting a diagnosis and cure in order to legitimate their experience of feeling unwell. Yet often what individuals experience are the disabling effects of an illness which may elude any classification, obvious diagnosis or cure. This points to the problematic nature of clear classification systems based only on organic criteria, which reflect traditional reductionist ways of thinking, and which are an outcome of purely scientific understandings of truth (Malterud 1987a, 1987b).

Concerns about this process of medicalisation led Richard Zaner (cited in Toombs 1988:200) to clarify the position of the body within illness as one of 'perilous equivocation':

> On the one hand it is a strictly biological organism; on the other it is the focus of clinical diagnosis and intervention and as such it is not merely biological but also experienced by the person whose body it just happens to be.

Illness, disease and medicalisation

For individuals who are sick, the experience of illness poses many dilemmas. Their families and carers can become involved in the experience along with various health professionals. While it is assumed that illness and disease are companions, this is not necessarily so. However, as Malterud(1987a:206) has argued 'disease is neither sufficient or necessary to explain illness'. Some illnesses, despite being disabling, have no apparent underlying disease entity as discerned by contemporary testing techniques. And many diseases do not exhibit illness effects until the disease is advanced, for example hypertension and some cancers. Yet the health care culture relies on the scientific notion of cause and effect, which in turn depends on organised practices, protocols, language and social groupings determined by a scientific model of inquiry.

Where there is no obvious cause of an illness, medical management becomes difficult, in some cases impossible for the doctor, the western expectation being that doctors will diagnose and treat the underlying cause of disease. Unless the illness is accompanied by sense data, which can be verified through scientific means such as pathology or radiology, the only alternative explanation, and there has to be one for classification, is that the patient's condition is psychosomatic. Worse, the patient can be labelled a 'malingerer'.

Along with the necessity to find a causal link for disease, scientific method is reliant on categorisation and decontextualisation. Medicine classifies diseased bodies into categories which order bodies into physiological systems, which are then collapsed into a number on the computer data base. Hospitalisation perpetuates this categorisation, potentially leading to an objectification of the individual undergoing the personal experience of the illness or disease. The person's physical body, in other words, becomes the focus of attention and care while their subjective experience of illness is ignored.

Malterud explicates the apparent pitfalls of this process, in particular the shift to emphasising diagnosis as the goal of management resulting in an 'endless succession of medical investigations' (Malterud 1987a:207). The recent move to grouping patients under Diagnosis Related Groups (DRGs) for funding purposes raises similar concerns regarding categorisation and decontextualisation.

The point here is not that knowledge of disease processes and treatment is unimportant, but that during illness the person experiences a dysfunctional body rather than a disease process. Individuals suffering various disorders understand their experience(s) from the changes in bodily function, in their lifestyle and how they are perceived by friends and colleagues. Their interactions with the world are changed, often permanently and thus their perceptions of self are changed. The underlying biological cause, while pertinent for treatment, is often irrelevant to the daily life of the individual who needs to revise his/her place in a world whose parameters have shifted because of the individual's changed capabilities.

While nurses also work within a schema of medical categorisation, their practice requires them to be more aware of the way in which individuals make sense of such experiences. This is because nurses deal daily with the human experience in illness and disease, with the intimacy of the body and with preparing for rehabilitation or death. They are unable to avoid such interfaces. Nurses work closely with the body, during which they perform actions that require vigilance about potential disruption to the individual's embodied self. This nursing vigilance is displayed in ways which include language, gesture and bodily positioning by the nurse who attempts to put the patient at ease during the procedure. Patients identify these actions as the nurse demonstrating respect for them (Beech & Norman 1995).

Nurses also are required to 'read' the body, interpret responses accurately and respond appropriately in their practice with patients. The difference between nursing and medicine, in this sense, inheres in nursing's more central concern with human experience, whereas medicine is more centrally concerned with the disease process (Pearson 1984, Watson 1988, Lumby 1992, Taylor 1994). While these different perspectives are complementary in terms of health care, the scientific framework of medicine works against such a gestalt through its privileging of disease over illness.

A disease centred orientation also continues to determine the political and financial structuring of health care, which in turn perpetuates the status quo in education, practice, legislation and research. Yet there is another side to this story of disease, and to explore this two nursing studies will be used later in this text. Personal and group narratives will illustrate the daily experience of women facing life and death because of their diseased bodies and subsequent liver transplants. Other studies addressing the way in which health professionals approach individuals from a gendered perspective are provided as further critique, while a variety of philosophical and historical positions regarding sex, gender and the body will be put forward.

Perspectives on the body, sex and gender

So what are the mediating influences historically and culturally which have determined our contemporary beliefs about bodies, sex and gender? 'It's a boy/girl!' are the initial words usually uttered at the birth of a baby. The sexing of individuals begins at the first moment of entry into the world (or even before that as we scan for signs of sexual difference in utero). And it is the genital organs which provide the initial information to the observers. This information is withheld until after the head and trunk are birthed (except in breach births) and so the sexing is delayed. The differentiation of gender into masculine and feminine through anatomical means was, however, not always so clear.

Anatomists such as Galen, in the second century, developed models showing that the reproductive organs of women were the same as men but 'their's [women's] were inside the body and not outside it' (Laqueur 1992:4). This belief, that there was only one sex, extended into the Renaissance period. An 'external' penis granted individuals higher status than those with an 'internal' penis. Characteristics such as being active or passive, hot or cold arose as necessary deviations of this gender binary that were also used for categorising individuals. In turn, social boundaries were thus determined. It was not until the 1700s when the vagina was actually acknowledged through naming that the notion of one sex was questioned. The increase in biological knowledge by the 1800s led to a plethora of texts arguing the difference between women and men, not only physically but also socially and morally (Jordanova 1989).

The very first question asked after a birth is 'what did you have?' reinforcing the importance of biological sex as a signifier of identity. Through their language and qualified responses during the birth, both doctors and nurses play an important part in reinforcing this sexing stage of birthing, while all other cultural discourses are also influential.

The body itself has been understood differently through history and across cultures. The privileging of reason and philosophy to the male has relegated the body to the 'other', that is the female, while science has, by necessity, used the body as object for much of its inquiry (Gatens 1991:122). This has rendered the body passive as well as relegating it to the 'unspeakable' because of its association with the 'dirty', the 'diseased' and with death. By association, women have also been identified with the everyday, ordinary things of life, the things which are not seen to contribute in any substantial way to cultural development. The notion of the body as dirty is perpetuated by medical discourse throughout the ages, hence those working with the body, particularly nurses, are perceived as doing 'dirty work' (Lawler 1991). The question here may be not that the body is gendered through illness but that the body itself is gendered through being relegated to the categorisation of 'healthy body' (male) or 'unhealthy body' (female) just as historically it had been categorised through notions of active/passive or hot/cold.

The mechanistic view of the body in medicine, the body-as-machine, has also encouraged a disembodied view of illness. Today, because of increased technology, pharmacological interventions, organ transplants and plastic surgery, this understanding of the body as controlled and controllable has been extended. The contemporary body can be transformed, re-figured and re-arranged. We even use the language of re-arrangement when speaking of cosmetic surgery and gender reassignment. Media messages tell us that we can recreate our bodies through diet, exercise and surgery. As a cultural medium, our bodies are also regulated by norms perpetuated through advertisements and images. In order to achieve the ideal body, research shows for example, that '80% of nine year old suburban girls [in the USA] are making rigorous dieting and exercise the organising discipline of their lives' (Bordo 1993:270).

Sex(uality) and gender

The terms 'sexuality ' and 'gender' are often used synonymously in everyday conversation. In medicine, genetic disorders are usually aligned with sex, reflecting the biological categorisation which is essential to the scientific view. The contemporary French theorist Michel Foucault in *The History of Sexuality Vol 1* (1984) argues that 'sex' is an effect rather than an origin and is produced by specific discursive practices. Sex is thus invested with meaning through certain discourses not disorders. Many illnesses are specific to either males or females, not only genetically, such as the sex-linked disorders, but also socially or epidemiologically because of the prevalence of certain diseases among one gender rather than the other. This linking of disease with certain genders is a mixture of historical medicalisation (such as hysteria and its alleged specificity to females), and cultural and environmental influences (such as spinal injuries among young males).

In distinguishing between sex and gender, Jordanova (1989) notes that while sexuality implies feelings, drives or actions, gender refers to the difference between masculine and feminine. Gender is a more inclusive category not necessarily involving sexual expression. Another distinction made by some theorists, particularly feminists, has been that gender is a social construction while sex is about physiological difference. Feminist philosopher Elizabeth Grosz (1994) claims that the majority of feminist theorists today would probably fit into this latter category of social constructionism, including Juliet Mitchell, Julia Kristeva and Nancy Chodorow.

The studies used in this chapter have been chosen not for their female-related disease prevalence (which relies primarily on the physical body as the organising schema) but because of the opportunity to offer women's perspectives on their experiences of illness, given the lack of gender specific clinical studies. The women in the two studies examined later claimed that the opportunity to share their stories allowed them critically to analyse predetermined sex differentiated cultural images and roles, which they had previously taken for granted. One such role was the apparent stereotyping by their general practitioners as women who were 'ordinary' tired mothers despite their deteriorating physiological status, which was quite 'extraordinary'.

Historical perspectives on gendering bodies

An exploration of the historical position of women and their bodies may explain the way in which women have experienced control socially and medically. Barbara Duden in her text, *The Woman Beneath the Skin*, reminds us that the body was only placed under medical scrutiny towards the end of the eighteenth century. Prior to this, the bodies of women were identified as magic and powerful because of the way they were seen as 'vessels of life and death' (Duden 1991:8).

After all their bodies housed the forces and substances that could produce good as well as evil: blood, the periodic flow, the afterbirth, the amniotic fluid and finally the 'mother' (womb) which like an oven could bring forth and take life (Duden 1991:8).

The regulation of women's bodies (viewed as polluted) was included in the training of Medieval saints (Duden 1991) while the Catholic Church today still attempts to control women's bodies through edicts concerning reproductive choice. During the Counter-Reformation, any power previously held with women, particularly midwives, was transferred to the Church, and women's bodies were defined and described as demonic and evil. Midwives and healers were burnt as witches during public displays in which their bodies were dissected. As medicine took over the role of the Church, the body became the object of the 'medical gaze' which dissected the body, objectifying it through an anatomical atlas (Duden 1991). The sick bed, rather than the person, became the site of 'scientific' observation (Foucault 1976:164).

The evolution of hospitals enabled bodies to be homogenised and categorised according to disease. Bodies in hospitals were also separated according to sex, resulting in male or female wards. Rather than an encounter between the patient and the doctor, medicine became a social institution with a 'collective consciousness'. The body was not only controlled by medical surveillance, it was also disciplined through social expectations. Social status was determined by the way in which individuals controlled their lives, habits and bodies and this was particularly so for women. As the 'objective' science of medicine gained a superior position over the mythical science of the spiritual within society, so physicians replaced priests in the social hierarchy. Absolution of the soul by the priest through confession was replaced by absolution of the body through medicalisation and surgery. Notions of immorality were reconceptualised through explanations of disease and cure. The doctor/patient relationship took over the 'regulative moral functions of religion' (Turner 1992), establishing the female body as uncontrollable through its increased tendency to diseases.

Thomas Laqueur argues that there was a shift during the eighteenth century from viewing the female body as merely having certain sexual organs, which were a less developed version of male organs (that is the phallocentric view), to a view that reinforced the notion of the female body as 'different'. This notion of difference arose for many reasons but one important determinate was the gendering of work roles which arose from the industrialisation and urbanisation of western society. This was explained scientifically in the late eighteenth century by the medical philosopher Cabanis (Laqueur 1992) who asserted that the differences in bodily structure between men and women were more to do with the roles naturally assigned to them than to do with issues of reproduction.

The move to industrialisation encouraged a differentiation of the public (workplace) from the private (home), and the valuing of the former over the latter. The emphasis on gender differences discouraged women from the workplace since the characteristics assigned to women emphasised their caring and domestic responsibilities. The appropriate roles for a woman included caring for children and the family, and being dependent on the male breadwinner (Gamarnikow 1978, Savage 1987, Abbott & Wallace 1990, Turner 1992). The explosion of medical and scientific knowledge along with the power this endowed to those with the knowledge of the mysteries of the body, meant that the functions and malfunctions of the body became the determinants of their gendered status as medicalised bodies.

During the nineteenth century, women were increasingly viewed and treated as 'invalids'. At this time the pathologist Rudolph Virchow claimed that a woman was 'a pair of ovaries with a human being attached' (Fausto-Sterling 1985:90). Between 1880 and 1910 because of the causal links made between potential sexual transgression by women and mental illness, surgical intervention was employed to reduce this risk. Clitoridectomy, circumcision and even castration (oophorectomy) were performed particularly as a means of controlling women who would not conform to social and cultural expectations of womanhood (Lovell 1981). After all, the family, the health of children and the moral guardianship of society all depended on women fulfilling certain roles and expectations (King 1992). These social expectations mediated the medical practices of the time. To be frail and of ill health was deemed to be the ideal state for women, conforming as it did to social and medical expectations. In 1870, a physician (cited in Lovell 1981:28) described the 'angelic' cancer victim thus :

> Suffering and agony have marbled that fair brow; pain and torture have sowed lilies where once were beds of roses, and the light of heaven gleams forth from the wondrous depths of those glorious orbs.

While the medicalisation of the body has extended to both genders, there is evidence that the female body has been labelled as pathological, requiring not only medical attention but often bed rest and isolation. Gendered images are used to portray illnesses, reinforcing the way in which medical discourse contributes to the gendering of society. Affective mood disorders such as depression and anxiety are still represented by passive female imagery in pharmacological advertisements while active male imagery is used for disorders which might limit strenuous activities, portraying the male as active in being able to overcome the disorder (Jordanova 1989). One of the main contributing factors here may be the complexities of the female reproductive stages. Today women are expected to see the doctor about what were previously normal events such as diagnosis of pregnancy, the various stages of pregnancy and the birth itself. When the birth does not go as planned, the doctor is often praised for his expert intervention.

This disease focus of western medicine has also meant that because women access the doctor about routine reproductive issues, such as painful menstruation, then women's bodies are continually viewed as 'sick', deviant or unhealthy. This is not a recent phenomenon. Gilman's (1973) experience of the 'rest cure' prescribed by S. Weir Mitchell, a neurologist, and which she described in her book, *The Yellow Wall Paper*, highlights the way in which the socio-political norms regarding gender were perpetuated by the medical profession's practices. In turn, these practices helped to reproduce the belief that women should be socially and medically controlled, silenced and made obedient for the sake of their own well being. As well, the economic benefit derived from constructing women as perpetual patients was clearly identified by a male physician in 1905 (Lovell 1981:29):

> The treatment of women has always contributed toward the yearly income of the general practitioner, while the gynaecologist continues to fatten upon the revenue he receives from operations. Ovarotomies and ... laparotomies have become an epidemic in some localities to the extent that many surgeons think they will be branded as being unskilful if they allow their patients to get well without operative procedures.

Childbirth was also reinterpreted through medical discourse, alienating it from what had been a normal part of life (as it still is in many countries without western medicine). With the introduction of technology into childbirth around the middle of the 18th century, predictability and control became part of the expectation of birthing. The employment of predictability and control in health care practice can be quite reassuring to contemporary mothers who often have roles in both private and public spheres but through this technological framework the maternal body was thus viewed as inviting complications that require medical intervention.

Just as the introduction of the dissection of corpses in the 18th century endowed the medical gaze 'with a plurisensorial structure' (Foucault 1976) thus altering the way in which disease and treatment was viewed, so the ultra scan has changed the way in which pregnancy is described and treated. An ultra scan is now routinely 'offered' to women thus refocusing the medical gaze from the 'spectacle' (Foucault 1976) of the woman's body to the interior, which previously had only been accessible as a corpse. The invisible (the interior) is now immediately visible to the doctor via the scan, thus granting even more access to the processes of intervention. It is still the doctor as the masculine viewer who lifts the veil of science, who reads the scan for the potential parents and who therefore becomes the seer, the one who knows (Jordonava 1989).

Likewise it is the doctor who listens, sees, feels and reads the surface of the body and interprets the results of the various tests. This aligning of medicine with privacy and power continues even today where medical texts, notes and images are not freely available or accessible to the public, either because of the language used or because the content of the text is regarded as not 'appropriate' for others to view. Despite the rhetoric of informed consent and patient centred care, patients are still denied access to their clinical data, leading to the conclusion by Jordonava (1989:137) that '...both medicine and science bear ambivalent relationships to the public realm socially, culturally, professionally and ideologically'.

The ability to view the growing foetus via an ultra scan also transfers the focus from the 'mother as patient' to the 'foetus as patient' potentially reconfiguring the pregnant woman as incubator. This notion of autonomy of the foetus is a central issue within the abortion debate. Today in most western societies, ultra scans during pregnancy have become routine while caesarean births are 'normal' birthing options, particularly in the USA. In 1980 Merchant reported that, in the USA, more than 1 million caesareans are performed each year (Merchant cited in King 1992:2). This is not to ignore the positive outcomes which have occurred because of medical and technological advances in pre and post natal care but to critique the way in which such advances have themselves become the controlling force in the discourse of reproduction. Meanwhile the woman is situated within an 'ideological web', which 'grants physicians the prescriptive control of the use and interpretation of reproductive technology' (King 1992:5). What was once hidden from view is no longer a mystery. And as in many scientific discoveries, a demand is created which gradually evolves into expected and accepted practice.

More recently, menopause has been colonised by medical terminology, labelling, and treatment. The typical signs of menopause — backache, headache and hot flushes have been configured as symptoms of a disease, which has become a multimillion dollar industry. A previously taboo subject, menopause is now spoken of openly, it is the focus of public debates, popular press articles, and multinational drug trials. It has gained respectability and can not only be spoken of but is actively encouraged as a topic for dinner conversation. MacPherson (1981:95) reassures us that despite the fact that 'no female function has been so degraded, dreaded and unmentionable as this final phase of the reproductive cycle...it is a natural biological event and is experienced universally by women'. MacPherson (1981:96) claims that 'the transformation of menopause into a disease has been a gradual collective and political achievement rather than the inevitable product of the natural evolution of society'. Menopause as a natural event not requiring intervention has disappeared. Meanwhile women are caught between the mediating influences of science, medical practice and everyday routine, attempting to negotiate the complex terrain of language, categorisation and professional control.

Women's experience of life threatening illness

The experience of a group of critically ill women at the interface of science, health care practice and illness is offered here as a glimpse of how these women managed their living while facing death. The collective stories of these women reflect the influence of their roles as women on their journeys through illness. The processes used in the studies, as well as the experience of facing death, encouraged a questioning of many assumptions about their bodies as gendered, reflecting the way in which the body is inscribed socially and culturally. The main themes that were explored had emerged from an earlier initial doctoral study (see Lumby 1992) and included:

1   control (which was the central issue);
2   the importance of relationships;
3   the element of spirituality which enabled a 'living with faith and hope';
4   body and bodily meanings;

5 preparing for both life and death and;
6 roles and needs as mother, wife and daughter.

Such revelations were reinforced in postdoctoral work in which the same illness experience was followed over two years with a group of women. The issue of control once more took a central position for these women. Issues relevant to the women in both studies will be discussed in the following passages and supported by theoretical positions.

The importance of control and power

As the central emerging theme for the women, control incorporated several elements. These included 'being in control', 'being out of control' and 'being controlled by others' from diagnosis through surgery and even after discharge. Women involved in both studies spoke of attempting to be in control of their illness and the subsequent experiences related to such a life threatening illness as end stage liver disease. They managed this control in a variety of ways, such as preparing for the smooth conduct of their households when they were either too ill to continue in their roles as main housekeeper, when they were in hospital or if they died. Many who had careers outside the home continued to work until they were quite debilitated. One woman who believed that she only had a prolonged virus, continued to work as a nurse up until her transplant. One night while preparing a birthday meal for her son after work, she felt so ill that she went to bed where her husband later found her comatosed from liver failure. By the next afternoon she had a new liver, although it was days before she knew about it. During the study she admitted that she had been feeling extremely ill but the wards were short-staffed and she believed that she could work through it. Her son's birthday then took priority over her illness.

This prioritising of families over illness was evident in all the stories of the women. One woman whose daughter was in her final year at school, placed her in a boarding school (much to the daughter's delight) mainly to protect the daughter from seeing the mother's deterioration. This woman also reorganised the roles of the older two daughters well before she was unable to cope, so that family life could proceed uninterrupted. Another one whose daughter was competing in a national event on the day of the mother's transplant, begged the daughter to go, claiming she wanted her to bring her home a trophy (which she did). One woman spoke of setting goals for herself in order to have a sense of control, while others planned their funeral services or celebrations in case they did not survive the transplantation.

During the initial doctoral study, Maree, the woman involved, spoke of how, during her first liver biopsy, she felt out of control and was left feeling powerless. She identified a range of issues which contributed to this, for example not being introduced to the staff. As she said 'they knew my name...I was labelled but they did not have name tags on' (Lumby 1992:151). When the doctor performed the procedure incompetently she felt 'out of control' because choice had been removed from her and when he spoke to another doctor across her body as if she was not present, she felt like a 'lump of meat'. The nature of her diagnosis and prognosis made this experience even more unsettling since each investigative procedure was vital for accurate diagnosis and subsequent treatment. From that time on Maree was determined to take control. She insisted on becoming part of any decision making, gaining information at all stages of her disease process. This meant that she turned her feeling of lack of control, of 'fear and horror' to a feeling of 'preparing for battle'. Because of her insistence on being kept informed, she was labelled a 'difficult' patient. As she became more debilitated she developed further strategies to control her fear. 'I thought only of the now, not a couple of hours ahead. I put my energies into what is happening now and not into the future. When I reflect, it is in retrospect , not in anticipation' (See Lumby 1992:154).

As a result of regaining control, after she received the call that a liver was available, she felt 'self -ufficient'. Like all the women in the study, she believed that she would survive. Post-operatively, when she woke connected to a ventilator and a variety of invasive monitoring devices, she soon learned to remove the pulse meter from her finger which activated an alarm. Staff responded to this and once more she felt in control in the intensive care environment, an extremely controlling context for all patients. To establish equal control with the medical staff she always sat up and insisted on shaking their hands when they arrived at the bedside. This enabled her to gain level eye contact, which she perceived as reducing any potential power imbalance of either a patient/doctor or able bodied/disabled body/nature.

Maree's sense of losing control returned after discharge when she attempted to return to a work position commensurate with her previous abilities and seniority. She was identified as a 'liver transplant' and felt powerless once more. She felt trapped and made the connection between her past of being trapped in an abusive marriage with her present position of being trapped professionally (which she never had been). After conquering the disease, this situation seemed even more difficult for her to comprehend. Her father and brothers attempted to make decisions on her behalf and to direct her future which made her feel angry rather than grateful. She even viewed this as 'mind control' which was worse than the physical control she had felt prior to the transplant. In reflecting on her anger, she realised that this episode reminded her of the many times she had felt 'inadequate and stupid' as a young girl and a married woman (Lumby 1992:159).

During this initial study, Maree's personal story illuminated why a sense of control was so important. Although research that involved the group of women did not allow the same indepth critical analysis that had been possible with Maree, similar sentiments were expressed. Maree's personal story involved living in a family in which males dominated the decision making and the power. She understood this family dynamics in a new way as contributing to situations through life where she felt easily 'put down by men'. Her father was a well-known doctor and her two brothers were very large physically, as was her father. While their physiques as males were highly valued in society, her large physique as a woman was not. She claimed that she always felt ashamed of her body shape and size. Comparing herself to the social stereotype of the 'ideal' woman she found her image wanting. Maree was continually chastised for eating, as she was 'too big'. Later Maree reflected that 'big women find it harder to climb into areas of power because they are seen as aggressive, whereas smaller women do not have the same problem' (Lumby 1992:186). When she lost a lot of weight during her illness she spoke of feeling 'sexy' for the first time because her thin body image was that which society links with 'sexy' women. Meanwhile Maree perceived her brothers as being rewarded for their large frames.

Embodied, gendered experiences of illness

Body and bodily meanings were identified as important by the women in both studies. While they discussed their physical symptoms such as itchy skin and tiredness and their physical signs such as yellowed skin and clay coloured stools, they spoke and acted according to changing functions. Their lives were determined by the abilities of their bodies as they moved through various stages of deterioration. But they did not perceive their bodies as disabling their lives. Rather, they adjusted their lives to account for their physical deterioration because they appeared to identify self with the way in which they could interact in the world. It seemed that their self-worth came from their actions in the world and they went to great lengths to remain connected to the everyday world which they had become part of — the world that knew them as worthy in their own right and not just as diseased bodies.

At all times, for Maree, her body was herself. She did not exist as a person outside or separated from her body. Her body made her the person she had become even when she was healthy. During her deterioration, Maree spoke of herself in terms of size and gender because she had always felt that her size had 'denigrated' her as a female. She had not ever felt truly 'feminine', which she understood to be related to bodily shape and weight, expensive clothes, accessories and attention to hair, all of which held no interest for her. She alluded to herself in terms of food and/or power. When she was forced to increase her calories after her transplant, she spoke lovingly of this time as the first in which she had been 'encouraged' to eat. Prior to this, her experience of food was that it was forbidden to her. But at all times her body was herself. Her yellowed skin and severe weight loss signalled to the outside world that she was unwell. She also developed dark circles under her eyes and moved listlessly. But the 'true' signs were hidden, known only to Maree. These were the clay coloured stools and bright yellow urine as well as the severe itch which increased in severity. She was also aware of the deteriorating blood tests used as a criterion for determining transplantation.

Maree attempted to control her deteriorating body by resting for long periods and then undertaking a task around the home such as pruning the hydrangea, which she maintained as a semblance of normality. When asked why she needed to do this she replied that it was the time to prune them and since she looked after the garden it needed to be done. Maree lived throughout the illness in an embodied way in which she gradually adapted to a less active role. This was highlighted after surgery when Maree 'wondered what was missing' until she realised that her body 'itch had gone' (Lumby 1992:177). It was as if she had grown with her changed body and when her body returned to its previous state she no longer recognised it.

Several women did find their physical changes quite concerning during their illness but this appeared to be linked with their previous self-image. One of the women, who was previously petite, spoke of how she hid her body through clothing as she began to retain large amounts of fluid. After their transplant, all the women found the increased weight from cortisone treatment to be an ongoing battle particularly if they had been slim all their lives. It seemed, for some women, that appearance took precedence over prognosis in terms of concern.

Maintaining normal roles and protecting others

The women identified their roles and needs as mothers, wives and daughters as a central focus during their illness because of the way in which this impacted on their experience. Even up to and during the night of the transplant, Maree continued her nurturing role, comforting and reassuring her daughters, her parents and her brothers. She spoke individually to each of her three daughters telling them of her love for each one and her hopes for their futures. She continued to meet her husband's needs although he seemed unable to meet hers. She even spoke minimally about the transplant to her parents despite her own need to talk. This was in an effort to protect them. While she shared experiences with her eldest daughter, she did not speak openly with the other two (who on interview spoke of their resentment regarding this). Her rationale for this was one of protection.

The other women told similar stories of protection, keeping things as normal and balanced as possible both at home and at work and hiding their deterioration from friends, family and colleagues. This appeared to be linked to where they felt valued, that is in the public or the private sphere. Maree, valued in her professional role as an expert clinician, worked for as long as possible, while others maintained their involvement in the day-to-day management of the home which was a social expectation of these women whose mean age was 40 years. While this may be different for younger women today because of changed expectations regarding gendered roles, social and cultural structures and images still appear to create divisions between the way in which boy's and girl's roles are mediated even during their schooling (Foster 1996).

Despite increased social debate and action concerning the gendering of roles, women are still regarded as the main nurturers in the private domain, and for nurses this extends to the public (or is it private?) domain of health care. The linking of gender and the physiological characteristics of the body with certain roles in society is seen in much of the research regarding role differentiation and work.

Scientific inquiry into the workplace, until 1986, concentrated on the female reproductive system at the expense of the male reproductive system (Kenney 1986). These studies claimed women were 'vulnerable' in terms of work which served to keep them out of certain jobs. The outcomes of such research leave the male body privileged over the female body in terms of certain work, despite the fact that women carry children to term while working full-time, often in rice fields or factories, as well as undertaking the household tasks which can be more demanding than the male workplace in terms of heavy work. The women in these studies did not reveal themselves to be vulnerable in their roles — rather, the contrary was the norm.

Trusting the doctor

Trusting the doctor — the priest of science — also emerged from the studies. Doctors' legislated and accepted roles in diagnosis, treatment decisions and referrals have ensured that they continue to make the major decisions relating to illness and disease, including the type of discourse surrounding the gendered illness experience. Two women told stories of the trust they had invested in their general practitioners of twenty years despite obvious deterioration in their conditions. These stories also reflected the way in which the women were placed in gendered categories by these doctors.

One story concerns a woman who continued to feel so tired that she spent the day lying down while her children were at school and only got out of bed when they returned home. This went on for almost ten years. When she mentioned this extreme lethargy to her general practitioner, he told her that she was just a 'normal mother' who needed a vitamin B injection. This woman, with a past history of hepatitis B, spoke of getting thinner and thinner with a spleen like a football. When she started to have nose bleeds her general practitioner blamed her for picking her nose.

The second story concerns a woman who also experienced extreme tiredness. Various doctors she consulted blamed the tiredness on her having 'too many' children. This highlights the position of trust which doctors enjoy in our communities because both women accepted the explanation given. It may also highlight the way in which mothering has been constructed socially with certain expectations of normal and accepted states of being associated with this role, for example extreme tiredness.

Recovering their embodied selves and roles

After recovering from their initial transplant, most of the women in the studies spoke of the change in themselves as individuals and therefore in their roles as women. Because they had faced life and death and taken control, they were changed and determined to take control of their future in ways which their families did not always understand or accept. While they were changed by the experience, the families had not changed in the same way; thus the women were expected to get on with their prescribed 'private' roles of being mothers, wives and daughters.

Maree and the other women spoke of feeling guilty about living their lives in a more selfish way, which they interpreted as giving oneself more time as an individual. Inherent in this was being guilty about meeting one's own needs because mothering was about nurturing others. Maree also spoke of how the practical everyday things are left to women. Any disruption of this is unacceptable to the family who may have to pick up some of these roles.

Because of her traditional family, Maree's change was even less acceptable. She spoke of the effect it had on family dynamics: 'The children have noticed it...my parents are concerned about it...my husband is denying it' (Lumby 1992:187).

The way in which the women actively sought out other women for support during their illness was also an interesting issue arising from both studies. All the women spoke of receiving help from their female friends who understood their concerns. While the women spoke of particular individuals as being supportive or non-supportive during their experience, Maree had organised what she called her 'Circle of Relationships'. These were all women whom she had known and trusted over her lifetime as a nurse, mother and wife. Some were in the country and others close by, but she was very clear about the way in which she linked with each woman. By building up a network Maree believed that she was not overloading any one person. When the nights were long during her wait for her donor liver, she would ring those women who were on night duty in the country and talk to them.

She was active in her development of links with women and made a conscious effort to utilise these when appropriate. When she rang someone she did not want 'sympathy' but she wanted to be 'uplifted' even if that meant someone might 'pull me to pieces if they felt it necessary' (Lumby 1992:165). She also wanted to talk about her fears and to cry without being silenced. She believed that it was often easier to get support from outside the family because families are more likely to define needs from their understanding rather than the perspective of the person who is ill. In Maree's case her mother wanted to help by tidying drawers while Maree wanted to share how she felt. Other women spoke of how their mothers took over and tried to control their lives pointing out that control was not necessarily only from men.

Gendered embodiment and women's roles

Aligning women's health status with social problems and lifestyles also perpetuates an understanding of the female body as socially disordered. Because of the earlier scientific view that women had smaller brains than men anatomically (Lane 1990) there was an assumption that they were weaker physiologically and psychologically. Charlotte Perkins Gilman (1973), an early feminist writer, was admonished by her physician for reading and writing since he believed that this was the cause of her 'feeble' mind. Despite this, Perkins Gilman went on to be a prolific writer, her career interspersed with periods of 'melancholia'. Her writings reveal her desperation to find time to write between children, domestic chores and a domineering husband whom she did not love. This desperation for self-fulfilment, for a career of one's own outside the home is still experienced by women but the difference now is that these experiences are publicly debated and somewhat supported institutionally by maternity leave and child care.

While not yet entirely accepted by those who continue to identify women as the primary child carers, there are presently enough women undertaking careers while birthing and bringing up children to provide support for women to be involved in a full-time career during and after motherhood. Perhaps today Gilman's melancholia would not have been diagnosed as resulting from the overtaxing of her feeble mind. Instead, she could have hired a full-time nanny and written daily because she was rich.

The contemporary problem is that many women identify and accept that they have two major jobs, one as homemaker/mother and one as full-time worker outside the home. This is backed by recent research from the Australian Institute of Family Studies (Horin 1995). The outcomes of this research shows that, rather than participate in the work in the home, men prefer their female partners to reduce their working hours outside the home to part-time work in order to provide a more stable and 'nurturing' home environment. The researchers concluded that 'despite public and private protestations of egalitarianism, it was overwhelmingly mothers who provided the solution to balancing work and family roles' (Horin 1995:1). While men continue to dominate the public space and ignore the private in this way, women will be unable to find a sphere where the two spaces can merge to ensure a better balance is found not by women but by society.

Domination of the female body

This history of domination of the female body has left a legacy which appears difficult to address because of its complexity. The many hormonal phases of women's reproductive cycle continue to inform a large part of the research and practice of medicine. Scientific and medical discourse genders bodies and portrays the feminised body in terms of reproductive function and disease.

The medicalisation of the various stages of reproductive development has produced medical and surgical specialists and specialties, specialist education and research institutes, specialist pharmacological products for treatment and prevention, natural therapeutic modalities, specialised language and a plethora of texts along with weekly magazine articles which tend to sensationalise the everydayness of the various 'conditions' which women 'suffer'.

Recent research has highlighted a continuing lack of decision making by women when it comes to their bodies. King (1992) comments on the fact that today, during the care of the birthing woman, technology such as foetal monitoring, in vitro fertilisation and caesarean section distances the physician and the woman with the result that the person in the body is forgotten. In her place is a reproductive machine.

The question nevertheless arises: why do women allow this to happen? Why don't they insist on being part of an informed decision regarding their bodies? Other areas being debated in the 1990s include the use of hormonal replacement therapy during and post menopause, breast reconstruction, liposuction, facelifts and other interventions loosely described as 'plastic surgery' (Seaman & Seaman 1977, Orbach 1989). Perhaps studies concerning patient satisfaction may help to inform this apparently passive acceptance of the mediating influences of medicine and science on the feminised body.

In a study of patient satisfaction with intern performance, female patients showed greater satisfaction with their interns' work than did the male patients. Controlling for demographic variables and the gender of the intern, this positive rating by women remained consistent for most of the measurements of patient satisfaction. While overall satisfaction by both men and women was linked to their interns' biomedical competence and ability to communicate, women tended also to 'weigh a personal dimension' (Lieberman, Sledge & Matthews 1989:1827). The latter dimension related to items involving concern for the person, courtesy, availability and bedside manner. In contrast, the male patients' satisfaction with performance emphasised the importance of active dialogue by the intern regarding their condition. The results of this study may be read in the light of Gilligan's work (1988), which showed that because women value interpersonal relationships more than men, they may also minimise dissatisfactions and concerns in an effort to reduce conflict and confrontation.

There is evidence that those patients who present with health concerns not explicable through pathological findings are mainly women (Malterud 1887a, 1987b). In two separate studies, Malterud (1987a, 1987b) found that health problems in female patients often confused the general practitioner because they were classified as 'unspecific' or 'various' and so they did not fit into any disease classification. The influence of cultural and social standards on presentation of health complaints and behaviour in the 'sick' role has been shown to make a difference to the way in which women behave.

Despite the lack of scientific evidence of disease in 122 case studies in Malterud's work, through the use of a process named the 'clinical communicative method', women patients were found to be perfectly competent in providing an explanation of their undefined illness if the doctor-patient communication was appropriate. The basic problem appeared to lie with the way in which practitioners communicate in a gender specific way. Listening to the woman and allowing her to utilise her own 'medical' description were methods that improved the doctors' insight.

While there is some evidence that the attitudes of both sexes to female patients is seen as negative, female physicians allocate female patients more surgery time than their male counterparts. Professionals involved in mental health therapy have also been shown to be biased when it comes to their view of women. While the 'mature healthy socially competent man' in a study was rated against with the 'mature, healthy, socially competent individual', the 'mature, healthy, socially competent woman' was described as lacking, submissive, conceited about her appearances, easily influenced and hurt, emotional and excitable (McBride and McBride 1982).

Research on gender: what does it tell us?

The scientific research on women's experiences has tended to focus on women's bodies as 'diseased' (Dunbar et al 1981) and research on women's health issues has predominantly been directed to using women as 'subjects'.

researchers have moved to understand women's experiences of health and illness through methods such as narrative inquiry, which illuminates other factors that cause dis-ease in lives as well as bodies. Critical issues for women include such experiences as the complexity of birthing children and raising them while also being the 'good' daughter to ageing parents, the 'good' wife to an often absent husband, the 'ideal' employee, the 'perfect' mother, community worker, housekeeper, cleaner, cook and moral guardian. Such research and the qualitative methods used have, however, been viewed as invalid and the outcomes easily ignored within the scientific world where decisions about health care are made.

Nurses have also neglected the area of gendered research in the past although this appears to be slowly changing. Similarly, there is little research which explores whether nurses either assume gender as a natural category or deny its importance as a factor in illness.

Comparative studies which examine men and women's experience of the same illness are also scarce. Low (1993) explored the recovery of women and men from myocardial infarction and coronary artery bypass surgery. The study highlighted differences in recovery times and quality of life between men and women. Women appeared to have more difficulty in recovering from an infarction or bypass graft, however such results were qualified by the measures used and the lack of data on psychosocial factors. There is some evidence that women receive less aggressive treatment for coronary artery disease and that onset of the disease is later in women; but even with this accounted for, several studies have shown that women spend more days in bed following bypass surgery and experience more emotional difficulties (Stanton cited in Low 1993).

It is unclear what role affective variables such as anxiety and low efficacy play in this delayed recovery. Another suggestion was that women adopt the 'sick' role more readily, however it is also acknowledged that perhaps women are more open than men about their symptoms, their fears and their functional ability.

There is also some data suggesting that while women do not return to work as soon as men after bypass surgery, they take up housework at home earlier than men. This highlights the gender bias of some research, in particular the inadequacy of using 'return to work' (meaning work in the public sphere) as a variable to assess quality of life and recovery in patients after infarction and/or surgery.

While it was assumed that the increasing number of women in medicine would somehow change the culture of medical practice, there is little evidence that this is the case. The research investigating differences in the ways in which doctors interact with men and women patients is mixed. A study by Mendez, Shymansky & Wolraich (1986) showed that female doctors deal with the affective aspect of their interactions with patients more effectively than males and this is corroborated by other studies (Mehrabian 1972, Mehrabian & Ksionzki 1974), which indicate that female doctors are more able to convey distressing information with sensitivity, compassion and respect. This aspect of care is of considerable interest to medical educators who wish to encourage this component of medical practice in medical curriculum. Female doctors were also influential in reducing patient anxiety during pelvic examination of young adolescent girls aged 12–19 years (Seymour et al 1986). While having undergone a previous pelvic examination appeared to reduce anxiety during examination if a semi-sitting position was used, nevertheless examination in a supine position elicited high levels of post-examination anxiety in these adolescents when performed by a male physician. Such studies need further replication and application of results to everyday medical and nursing practice if we are to use research as a base for our practice.

With increasing numbers of women entering the field, however, it is becoming clearer that the gender of the doctor does not necessarily determine sensitivity to gender-based issues in health care. Comparative studies of male and female residents' attitudes and behaviours have shown that in the area of obstetrics female residents are less tolerant of women who are noisy, anxious or 'out of control' during the birthing (Zambrana, Mogel & Scrimshaw 1987). This was in contrast to the female doctors' voiced motivation for entering this area of specialty because female residents had claimed that they wanted to work with women in collaborative ways. Alternatively, male residents claimed that economics was their main motivation for moving into obstetrics yet their behaviours appeared to reflect a different story.

Social science's contribution to gendered research

Social scientists appear to have either ignored the issue of gender or worked within the scientific framework of biological categories concerning gender. Frequently, social scientists have studied only male subjects and extrapolated the results to women without questioning whether the criteria, methodology or aims of the study were gendered. Examples include past studies on cholesterol and alcoholism. Studies to do with alcoholism have focused on men to the extent that until 1980 only three studies out of 374 included females as subjects (McBride & McBride 1982) yet the results were used when treating women. This approach has now been questioned.

Perhaps the work which publicly highlighted the unscientific nature of gender biased research has been Gilligan's (1988) research on moral development. Finding discrepancies between her studies of girls' moral development and that of Kohlberg's (cited in Gilligan 1988) studies she began to investigate his original study from which he claimed that girls were behind boys in their stages of moral development. Kohlberg's study had only used boys as subjects and extrapolated the outcomes to girls who were then found to be 'behind' the boys. As Gilligan points out, the differences between males and females, when it comes to how they relate to the world and to others, particularly during their developing years, appeared to have been overlooked. The biased nature of his all-male population should have made Kohlberg's (cited in Gilligan 1988) research invalid because his stages of moral development had been developed from the social reality of only half of society.

Utilising Haug's memory work methodology with adult women and men, Crawford et al (1992) reinforced Gilligan's work demonstrating that many of our emotions are constructed with reference to justice and responsibility. While men expect they will be looked after, women are expected to be the ones who do the 'looking after'. Men, on the other hand, identify that it is their responsibility to make the world a 'just' place in which to live. While an ethic of responsibility and an ethic of justice have been identified as the two aspects of morality, the latter is privileged over the other and is more often than not identified with the male. Once more the woman is constructed as inferior just as girls were when measured using Kohlberg's moral development scores.

In traditional psychological research, the use of only males as subjects has been quite extensive, indeed expected and accepted with minimal critique. Convenience sampling was used historically since all-male populations were easily accessible in jails or medical schools. There is still evidence of gender bias in contemporary research, mainly through the continued use of questionnaires designed over a decade ago. For example, the acknowledgment of men's work is used as a standard variable in family studies with no similar acknowledgment of women's work outside the home.

While it is arguably valuable for practitioners to understand illness experience from both a male and female perspective, it is equally important to note that research, which takes account of women's experience, may perpetuate a view of women as somehow aberrant or 'other'. This type of research has also been critiqued as poor research if there is no rationale for sorting into categories. The claim is that sorting needs to be done at the end of research after results demand the need to identify the 'why' of difference identified. Sorting at the beginning is said to cause bias by the researchers or bias within the methodology if women and men are treated differently. More recently the critique of such traditional methodologies and constructs of gender has led feminists to search for new methods, new theories and indeed new paradigms (Crawford et al 1992), which find a space for women's voices (Grosz 1990).

Nursing's dilemmas: towards a summary

Given the pedagogical confusion in which they appear to have practised historically, how can nurses reinterpret their roles from within their own paradigm? Or have they a vested interest in maintaining the scientific culture in which they work? Scientific practices divide people on the grounds of their biologically determined sex, and they privilege investigation of the disease above understanding the illness experience. Routines are often tailored to the needs and wants of the health professionals over and above that of the patients. And there is evidence that objectification of patients enables a distancing by professionals, which reduces their feelings of vulnerability. A scientific framework of practice assists this distancing.

Nurses claim that this framework prevents them from adopting flexible practices, autonomous decision making and patient centred care (Lumby 1995). They feel caught within a centrifuge of demands from colleagues, which prevents them from working with patients in the way they know best serves the patients' needs. In order to overcome this dissonance, many nurses adopt subversive tactics. Examples of this include challenging or ignoring routine medical orders if the patient appears to be suffering as a result of such orders, or prioritising patient comfort and safety above issues of efficiency, such as early discharge to enable increased client turnover. Such differences in emphasis create power struggles and ethical dilemmas within institutions whose main goal is to provide effective patient care for the least cost.

Until recently, hospitals had gender specific wards. So it was that nurses spoke of working in a men's ward or a women's ward and spoke of the advantages and disadvantages of both. Some of this differentiation occurred because of the sex specificity of certain diseases or the fact that doctors were very specialised and preferred to have 'their' patients in one ward. Whatever the reason, it has become part of traditional nurse talk to speak about working with men or women (and their bodies) rather than with patients. And nurses are very clear about the differences in nursing either sex, although one must question how much disease pattern and culture impacts on such generalisations. There are several groups of patients who are treated as sex neutral. These include the 'elderly', the 'disabled' and the 'mentally ill'. For nurses in Australia, how much does our education, culture and place as a feminised profession and emerging discipline within a certain historical time dictate our attitude to the way we presently nurse groups of patients?

Feminist philosophical representations of the body

Contemporary feminist philosophy is concerned to challenge traditional philosophical notions of the body, of sex and of gender, so it may offer some insights for nurses and nursing. In particular, feminist philosophers are interested in how western philosophy is grounded in a mind/body split which privileges the mind in a way which has important consequences for our understanding of the body. In its simplest form, this problem might be understood as the separation of human beings into a sex- neutral mind and a sexed body.

The question of a sex/gender distinction, which has preoccupied feminists, has evolved from this binary. It concerns the relationship between the female body (sex) and the abstract properties which have been attributed to that body (gender) . While it is clearly impossible to do justice to the complexity of current debates on these questions here, it is worth sketching some of the key lines of argument which concern nursing's theory and practice. One of the major oppositions in mainstream feminist thinking about the body lies between egalitarian (or biologically determinist) feminists and social constructionists. While the former tend to see the female body, with its reproductive potential, as a limit to women's participation in the public sphere (and consequently to their ability to live and work with men as equals), the latter argue that the female body is simply a biological entity whose capacities and potentials have been (negatively) coded by a dominant patriarchal ideology.

As Elizabeth Grosz points out in her recent book examining the problem of the body/mind split. from a feminist perspective, neither of these positions transcends or even problematises the mind/body split. Rather, they naturalise it:

129

... like egalitarian feminists, social constructionists share several commitments including a biologically determined, fixed and ahistorical notion of the body and retention of the mind/body dualism. 'Political struggles are thus directed towards neutralisation of the sexually specific body (Grosz 1994:16–17).

Central to contemporary feminist debates in philosophy is the question of how to develop a theoretical position which is inclusive of the body; this is a problem that nursing is also addressing. The impasse between biological determinism and social constructionism has produced intense argument; and a variety of alternative positions has emerged sometimes collectively grouped under the rubric of 'difference' feminism. In a recent collection of essays dealing with this question, Elizabeth Grosz argues that they way forward for feminist theory lies in thinking beyond the biological determinist/social constructionist binary. Specifically, she identifies a range of feminist thinkers who have discarded liberal notions of equality to the 'right to consider oneself equal to another or reject the terms by which equality is measured and to define oneself in different terms' (Grosz cited in Schor and Weed 1994:91).

Grosz, like a number of contemporary feminist philosophers, is concerned to reposition the body from the margins of theory to the centre. Grosz (1994) understands the body as interactive with culture, as something which both acts and is acted upon. To explain this interaction, Grosz uses the metaphor of a Moebius strip — a three dimensional figure of eight which turns on itself, thus allowing a fluid movement between the inside and the outside and back again.

Research within a scientific framework

While philosophical theories, particularly those taken by feminist philosophers, raise questions for those caring for the bodies of women and men and offer other ways of understanding their workplace structures and practices, they are necessary but not sufficient for a change in this culture. Cultures such as health care are dependent on certain dominant discourses which determine what other discourses are valid and therefore whose voice(s) are heard and whose are silenced. A practical move to highlight gendered perceptions and practices is to increase research on women's experiences within paradigms which are acceptable to the dominant scientific paradigm. This is essential when it is realised that scientists rarely read or confer outside their own research frameworks.

Research that enables a space for women' s voices to be heard and the development of distinctly feminist theories and methodologies, which remove woman from the category of 'other' are equally important. Allen, Alman & Powers (1991) argue for the retention of 'woman' as category in analytic research but not in generative research. Generative research is that which generates or creates new information about women and therefore foregrounds aspects of their lives previously unnoticed. In this type of research Allen et al claim that gender is not a variable because it constitutes the activity under scrutiny within the study.

There is no specific method linked to this type of research that often involves surveys and experiments. Analytic research or inquiry, on the other hand, focuses not on subjects but on discourse, and involves analysing or deconstructing the way in which women are spoken about in our society. Because the research is identifying relationships of the discourse with the way in which gender has been constructed, it seems feasible to identify gender as an important factor. This approach offers a critical look at the mediating influences in society that determine the feminised body. It overturns the view that gender is stable over time, culture and space, offering a self reflexive rather than a linear approach to epistemological development. Feminists who have used this approach to deconstruct and reconstruct discourse concerning 'woman', include Adrienne Rich (1978) and Sandra Harding (1986). This approach helps to overcome some of the problems inherent in presupposing gender categories as natural.

In relation to scientific inquiry into the body, investigating the experience of individuals in various states of health and illness appears to offer an alternative account of the body from which to gain additional perspectives to those of disease oriented research. Such investigations are able to record the body as an active and interactive participant in the experience — the body as *lived*, rather than as object. This appears to offer more hope than studies which treat sex as a pre-given variable, an essential categorisation tool *a priori* to the study. Studies which do not make such assumptions often necessitate the use of methodologies outside the traditional scientific model used to investigate disease.

Conclusion

An understanding of the human condition, the ontological rather than the epistemological basis of knowledge, can best be explored within a framework that can take account of meanings and actions of the phenomena under scrutiny. Methodologies which incorporate an embodied approach to studying the illness experience include phenomenology, critical and feminist paradigms.

Founded on the principles of embodiment from a critical feminist perspective, the studies used in this chapter explored the 'lived' world of women facing a life threatening illness. These methods enabled the women and the readers to gain a critical awareness of the 'lived' (experienced) female body interacting within the world of illness, disease and health care. Such an awareness questions the presuppositions on which traditional conceptions of gender and the body are founded, opening up the possibility for questioning practices built on such presuppositions.

REFERENCES

Abbott P, Wallace C (eds) 1990 Social work and nursing: a history. In: Abbott P, Wallace C (eds) The sociology of the caring professions. Falmer Press, Basingstoke

Allen D, Alman K K M, Powers P 1991 Feminist nursing research without gender. Advances in Nursing Science 13(3):54

Beech P, Norman I J 1995 Patient's perceptions of the quality of psychiatric nursing care: findings from a small-scale descriptive study. Journal of Clinical Nursing 4:117–123

Bordo S 1993 Unbearable weight: feminism, western culture and the body. University of California Press, Berkeley

Crawford J, Kippax S, Onyx J, Gault U, Benton P 1992 Emotion and gender: constructing meaning from memory. Sage, London

Duden B 1991 The woman beneath the skin: a doctors' patients in eighteenth century Germany. Harvard University Press, Cambridge

Dunbar S B, Patterson E, Burton, C Stuckert G 1981 women's health and nursing research in women's health. Advances in Nursing Science 3:1–125

Fausto-Sterling A 1985 Myths of gender: biological theories about women and men. Basic, New York

Foster V 1996 (in press) Space invaders: barriers to equity on the schooling of girls. Allen & Unwin, Sydney

Foucault M 1976 The birth of the clinic: an archaeology of medical perception. Tavistock, London

Foucalt M 1984 The history of sexuality: an introduction. Random House, New York

Gamarnikow E 1978 Sexual division of labour: the case of nursing In: Kuhn A, Wolpe A (eds) Feminism and materialism Routledge, London, 298–320

Gatens M 1991 Feminism and philosophy: perspectives on difference and equality. Polity Press, Cambridge

Gilligan C 1988 In a different voice: women's conception of self and morality. Harvard Educational Review 47:481–517

Gilman C P 1973 The Yellow Wallpaper. The Feminist Press

Grosz E 1990 Philosophy. In: Gunew S (ed) Feminist knowledge: critique and construct. Routledge, London

Grosz E 1994 Volatile bodies: towards a corporeal feminism. Allen & Unwin, Sydney

Harding S 1986 The science question in feminism. Cornell University Press, Ithaca

Horin A 1995 Jobs and families: how mums cope. Sydney Morning Herald Thursday, 24 August, 1.

Jordanova L 1989 Sexual visions: images of gender in science and medicine between the eighteenth and twentieth centuries. University of Wisconsin Press, Wisconsin

Kenney S 1986 Reproductive hazards in the workplace: the law and sexual difference. International Journal of the Sociology of Law 14:393–414

King C R 1992 The ideological and technological shaping of motherhood. Women's Health 19(2–3)

Lane A J 1990 To herland and beyond: the life and work of Charlotte Perkins Gilman. Pantheon Books, New York

Laqueur T 1992 Making sex; body and gender from the Greeks to Freud. Harvard University Press, Cambridge

Lawler J 1991 Behind the screens: nursing, somology, and the problem of the body. Churchill Livingstone, Melbourne.

Lieberman PB, Sledge W H, Matthews D A 1989 Effect of patient gender on evaluation of intern performance. Archives of Internal Medicine 149:1825–1829

Lovell M C 1981 Silent but perfect 'partners': medicine's use and abuse of women. Advances in Nursing Science 3(2):25–40

Low K G 1993 Recovery from myocardial infarction and coronary artery bypass surgery in women: psychosocial factors. Journal of Women's Health 2(2):133–139

Lumby J 1992 Making meaning from a woman's experience of illness: the emergence of a feminist method for nursing. Doctor of Philosophy thesis, Faculty of Nursing, Deakin University, Geelong

Lumby J 1995 Mapping the world of the nurse. Faculty of Nursing, University of Sydney. Unpublished research

Malterud K 1987a Illness and disease in female patients I. Pitfalls and inadequacies of primary health care classification systems – a theoretical review. Scandinavian Journal of Primary Health Care 5:205–209

Malterud K 1987b Illness and disease in female patients II. A study of consultation techniques designed to improve the exploration of illness in general practice. Scandinavian Journal of Primary Health Care, 5:211–216

McBride A B, McBride W L 1982 Theoretical underpinnings for women's health. Women and Health, Spring/Summer 6:1–2

MacPherson K 1981 Menopause as disease: the social construction of a metaphor. Advances in Nursing Science 3(2):95–113

Mehrabian A 1972 Nonverbal communication. Aldine Atherton, Chicago.

Mehrabian A, Ksionzki S A 1974 A theory of affiliation. Lexington Books, Lexington.

Mendez A, Shymansky J A, Wolraich M 1986 Verbal and nonverbal behaviour of doctors while conveying distressing information. Medical Education 20(5):437–443

Orbach S 1989 Fat is a feminist issue. Arrow, London

Pearson A 1984 The essence of advanced nursing care is being there. Nursing Mirror, 5 September, 159(8):16

Rich A 1978 On lies, secrets and silence. Norton, New York

Savage J 1987 Nurses and gender. Open University Press, Milton Keyes.

Schor N, Weed E 1994 The essential difference: books from differences. Indiana University press, Bloomington

Seaman B, Seaman G 1977 Women in crisis in sex hormones. Bantam Books, New York.

Seymour C, Durant R H, Jay S, Freeman D, Gomez L, Sharp C Linder C W 1986 Influence of position during examination, and sex of the examiner on patient anxiety during pelvic examination. The Journal of Paediatrics 108(2):312–317

Taylor B 1994 The ordinariness of nursing. Churchill Livingstone, Melbourne

Toombs S K 1988 Illness and the paradigm of lived body. Theoretical Medicine 9:201–226

Turner B S 1992 Regulating bodies: essays in medical sociology. Routledge, London

Watson J 1988 Nursing: human science and human care. A theory of nursing. National League for Nursing, New York.

Zambrana R E Mogel W, Scrimshaw SCM 1987 Gender and level of training difference in obstetricians' attitudes towards patients in childbirth. Women and Health 12(1):5–24

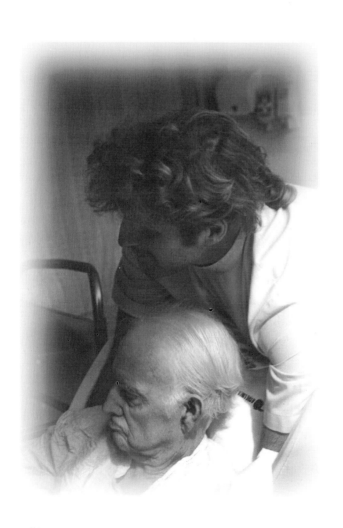

9

Masculinities, men's bodies and nursing

Stuart Newman

Introduction

A common theme in current literature on gender studies is that masculinity is in a time of significant challenge which some have described as 'crisis'. This 'crisis' for masculinity has emerged from the recognition that striving for the achievement of maleness and masculinity, as it is conceived, constructed and maintained in our society, is an extremely physically, psychologically and socially hazardous pastime for men. While contemporary feminism continues to show the adverse consequences of gender inequality and patriarchal systems for women, feminism has also been pivotal to the development of men's studies and a focus on masculinity.

Feminist 'attacks' on patriarchy have highlighted the need for men, as well as women, to be more critical of patriarchy because it is now recognised as our most powerful social convention, it is almost universal, but its (dis)advantages are questionable for both women and men and for society generally. While it is clear that men enjoy social and political advantage as a result of patriarchy, questions arise as to the value and nature of this advantage, particularly from physical, existential and embodied points of view for individual men and men as a group. In some ways, it is ironic to think that at one point being male in a patriarchal structure was the 'ideal position' and now there is cause to think otherwise.

This chapter focuses on the current thinking and debates surrounding masculinity, the construction and maintenance of masculinity in its hegemonic (patriarchal) form, and the inherent problems for men as they are compelled (in the social sense) to learn to live within the predetermined social rules that accompany the male role(s). The discussion traces the origins of these debates, the key issues that so far have been identified and speculates on how health care and nursing will and can feature in this emergent field.

Many questions are being addressed in the men's health agenda. However, it would seem that these questions are firmly based in the problems that the bureaucracy faces, in other words, the problems for the health care system, particularly in respect to men's access to and utilisation of services and the issues of morbidity and mortality among men. We are, though, starting to witness the emergence of literature that is taking into account the relationship between masculinity, its construction and maintenance in a patriarchal society and the problems for health care. We have, as yet, not systematically undertaken any detailed investigation into the notion of male embodiment, the experience of the lived male body as a healthy entity and how that relates to men's experience of illness, disability and disease. Clearly, this sort of investigation offers great benefits for clinicians in providing greater understanding about men's embodied experiences and how we might practise to take into account these experiences. From this standpoint, there are many issues for nurses and nursing that have not been addressed; this chapter is designed to stimulate and to focus attention on a poorly understood field.

Feminism, patriarchal masculinity and the notion of multiple masculinities

Contemporary feminism continues to campaign to undermine and deconstruct patriarchy — our most powerful social convention. The political feminist agenda is committed to eliminating gender based inequity and sexism because of the adverse consequences for women; and through their argument(s), feminist writers have 'been able to mount a profound critique of patriarchal society as an unjust system' (Horrocks 1994:1). For some men, it is likely that feminism can be frustrating because it creates indecision and apprehension about what they (as men) understand about what being male and masculine mean in a world where patriarchal advantage is under threat. It is not surprising that this indecision and apprehension exist, given the frenzied socio-cultural processes that have traditionally underpinned the construction of maleness and masculinity and which have helped the construct of men's 'comfort zones' about their masculinity viz. their social position, responsibilities, behaviour and sexuality.

In the wake of the deconstruction of patriarchy, the notion of patriarchal (hegemonic) masculinity is being subjected to increasing scrutiny and pressure. New questions are being asked not only by women but also by men, and these questions have unsettled the very foundations of what being male has come to mean and are challenging many traditional assumptions and beliefs about men and male role(s). Common cliches such as 'it's a man's world', endorse the argument that by virtue of their dominant position, men hold the social and political advantage over women. The overwhelming evidence from the literature illustrates that in such things as career paths, salaries and wages, payments for sporting achievements, and the public and private power men possess, the rewards have flowed to men. However, there are negative consequences of patriarchy that yet have not been systematically addressed and they relate to men's experiences.

The feminist 'offensive' against patriarchy has been a preponderant influence in the development of the view that patriarchal masculinity is in crisis. Feminism has caused us to acknowledge that patriarchy requires, creates and sustains a particular kind of masculinity, which supports the absolute functionalist process of ordering our society through a clearly defined and socially supported profile of acceptable male behaviour. This profile, which in turn is representative of the profile of patriarchy in general, has encouraged the development and articulation of the belief that the construction and maintenance of gender as we know it has adverse consequences, not just for women, but also for men and for relations between the sexes.

As a consequence of feminist work and, more recently, men's studies, it has become clear that while men may appear to hold the advantage over women, the social and political gains or benefits that result do not outweigh the physical, social and psychological and health costs incurred. Hearn (1994:47) strongly advocated that men must become involved in researching and writing on and about men because there is an absolute need for men to work practically and theoretically against patriarchy and to focus on men and masculinities as 'passionate players' in the process. He argues, citing Grosz (1987) that there is the need to do this in a critical way, 'not in the guise of the disinterested perspectiveless observer' because our knowledge will come from attempting to change the world and that this change will only come about from the adoption of a 'standpoint'. The concept of a standpoint for men's studies, as identified by Hearn, is more than taking a particular perspective — it is identifying the sources of social knowledge that grasp a unity between a social structure and its bearers, in this instance men. In this philosophical and epistemological sense, Hearn is taking a position similar to the feminist standpoint theory, yet men's studies does not entirely mirror feminism in its agendas.

For men, one of the greatest benefits of feminist and men's studies, has been the emergence of a new and extremely influential socio-political agenda surrounding masculinity. Fundamental to this agenda is the 'new wave' of the thinking surrounding men that includes the move away from a single incontrovertible notion of masculinity to the more expansive and emancipatory view of 'masculinities'.

Given the context in which hegemonic (patriarchal) masculinity has become institutionalised in our society, the idea of multiple masculinities is certainly problematic. In his book, *Masculinities and Identities*, Buchbinder (1994:1) argues that suggesting the idea of multiple masculinities twenty years ago would have been, to say the very least, 'quaint' and twenty years before that, most likely inconceivable, let alone tolerable. Masculinity has traditionally been seen as self-evident, natural, and, above anything else, the same in all contexts, not multiple and divided. Cornwall and Lindisfarne (1994:12), however, support the view of multiple masculinities and emphasised that the term 'masculinities' is not simply the plural of masculinity because masculinity is not a tangible unitary commodity nor is it an abstraction whose meaning is everywhere the same. Horrocks (1994), in his discussion of the idea of multiple masculinities, argues that it is a much more complex issue than some would have it. He suggests that while the concept of multiple masculinities represents greater latitude than that which exists within the traditional hegemonic framework, it does not necessarily mean that these masculinities are any less hegemonic. Rather, each society or culture creates and supports the masculinities it requires and is 'willing' to tolerate. In this sense, all shades of masculine identity ranging from macho to effeminate that are created through the use of the term 'masculinities' still serve to convey a common message; that men are not women. It is, as Horrocks would have it, that a male has to

> distance himself from femaleness and femininity, in order to prove that he is a male... . The masculine is the negation of the feminine, and this opposition varies from culture to culture... . What counts is not so much the content but the structural opposition between the two genders (1994:33).

While the debate continues, the adoption of the term 'masculinities', is a substantial move towards the establishment of a theoretical and political strategy in the attempt to deconstruct conventional stereotypes surrounding patriarchy and patriarchal masculinity and its workings and influences (Morgan 1992: 46).

Articulating maleness and masculinity: the problem of language

The sociolinguistics[1] surrounding masculinity contains many descriptive phrases for what constitutes being male. There are many examples that demonstrate how genderisation is embedded in our language and common forms of expression: 'boys don't cry', 'a man's got to do what a man's got to do' and, of course, the old favourite 'boys will be boys'! This sort of language has come to be symbolic of the traditional attempts to define maleness and masculinity that have been offered by so-called 'authoritative sources' and to a very great extent has come to reflect the socially 'correct' form.

Masculinity vis-a-vis femininity

The use of the terms, 'maleness' and 'masculinity', in common parlance is intrinsically problematic because it has become dependent upon the fundamental assumption that maleness and masculinity is not femaleness and femininity. Historically, accounts of masculinity depict it as antithetical to femaleness and femininity; that is, dichotomous logic has been applied here as in many other areas of our understandings of social order and human existences. Our inability to articulate maleness and masculinity is partly a result of a lack of language and the same applies to femaleness and femininity. The lack of language, however, does not mean we do not have a vocabulary of 'male words' or words that describe maleness and masculinity; the words work only as 'describers' and, as such, create the picture by which assumptions, beliefs and values are constructed. They do not, however, work to define the subject.

It is to this semantic problem that Gayle Rubin (1975:157–158) referred when illustrating the sex/gender system where, by virtue of sex (male or female), gender characteristics and suitable language are ascribed to males and females. The sex/gender system, according to Rubin, is semiotic[2] in nature because it assigns meaning to sexual difference and hence to the differential behaviours of women and men even, and in particular, in the absence of suitable language.

While the semiotic nature of the system can be recognised, it would seem that semiotics alone is an insufficient explanation. It is important to recognise or emphasise the powerful relational constructs that exist within the sex-gender system. It is the existence of these relational constructs that helps us to understand the symbols, signs and rules that accompany the masculine or feminine roles as they have been, and continue to be, constructed (Kimmel 1987:12). It is the semiotics and the relational constructs that create the relationship of sex to gender as binary in that the existence of one serves to give meaning to the other even if that meaning is only an understanding or an interpretation of what it is not.

The critique of a single dichotomous continuum (of masculinity/femininity) was extended by Friend (1987:31–32) who claimed that masculinity and femininity constitute disparate and autonomous sex-role identities rather than polar opposites on a single continuum. In other words, sex-role behaviours and attributes labelled as masculine and feminine constitute two separate continua. In relation to aligning masculinity and femininity on some dimension(s) of difference and/or similarity, diversity in sex-role identity can be viewed as occurring along a continuum about conformity to perceived sex-roles. Whichever the case may be, the important element is the recognition of the disparity that exists between maleness/masculinity and femaleness/femininity. In acknowledging this disparity, the essential factor is the associated politico/socio-cultural backdrop against which it is created, sustained and promoted that is the problematic and essential issue in any examination of masculinity. The acknowledged significance of the politico/socio-cultural setting in which masculinity is forged and maintained has been the impetus for many of the 'new' questions and has highlighted issues concerning maleness and masculinity. What remains problematic is that all this attention has focused on structural and socially organised elements as well as the way(s) in which women and men relate to each other in a particular socially ordered way. As yet, the debate has not systematically entered into or focused on how the subject 'male' is constructed and ultimately how men experience their masculinising and the subsequent outcomes of these experiences for themselves and others.

However, it is important to extend the discussion in this area because it is this antithetical view that initially served to establish the image of a continuum whereby what was masculine and/or feminine was neatly packaged (built on particular physical and embodied differences) and polarised at a socially 'suitable' distance. While this antithetical approach served some purpose, given the semantic problems identified, this polarisation can be interpreted in functionalist terms, to ensure the maintenance of the socially constructed and quite precise gender rule definitions and subsequent role behaviours. While this may well be the scenario, it can also mean it has simply been an attempt to camouflage the inherent difficulty in attacking the issues that inhere in constructs of masculinity, feminity, maleness and femaleness in a patriarchal and sex-differentiated society.

Competing accounts of maleness and masculinity

Perhaps because of our historical western scientific emphasis on categorisation and definition, we have experienced various attempts to explain or provide greater understanding of the issues surrounding maleness and masculinity; as a result, we have witnessed the rejection, revision and redefinition of a number of theoretical and conceptual frameworks. Consequently, we can identify transitional stages in the development of our understanding or current knowledge that have encouraged, and in some areas forced, alteration in our thinking and articulation of gender and the related issues.

Much of the earlier accounts of masculinity, from which later arguments evolved, were dedicated to discussion heavily influenced by 'naturalistic biologisim' as a pivotal means of explaining physical and embodied difference between women and men. A great deal of this investigation and literature is prescriptive and it equates biological substances (or lack thereof) with physical characteristics and ability (Brod 1987:184); hence it supports various sexual divisions within our society including divisions of labour and social roles according to the physical characterisation of sexual difference. The idea that maleness and masculinity are entirely genetically engineered and hormonally supported is a concept most contemporary gender researchers are unwilling to accept. There are some scientists who continue to argue the traditional view that deviation from the 'correct form' of masculinity, for example homosexuality, is or can be genetically linked; that efforts continue to seek scientific and genetic evidence for homosexuality raises questions about why this knowledge is sought. And recent media coverage on the reported discovery of a 'gay gene' has not resolved the debate but rather has fuelled it. The consequences of this knowledge for the health system and nursing are, as yet, unknown, but what is certain is that there will be consequences.

Only in the recent past have we moved away from conventional 'scientific wisdom' because of the recognition of the dominance and to a certain extent flawed nature of these highly explicit and detailed theories (Pleck 1987:21). Connell (1995:7) contends that the twentieth century has seen three main projects in the development of a science of masculinity. The first was based on clinical knowledge accumulated by therapists; the second was the development of social psychology and the notion of sex roles; and the third involves the recent developments in anthropology, history and sociology. However, as Connell further points out, traditional science may still have the edge in the argument about causal differences between men and women simply because of the perceived value of science and its influence in our society (1995:5). I suspect that in some circles this argument will continue, primarily because there is no conclusive explanation or causal relationship that satisfies those who seek 'hard' scientific evidence or 'proof' to account for gender issues or issues that appear to be genetically (biologically) determined, for example, aggressive behaviour in men.

Clinical knowledge accumulated by therapists enhanced the influence of psychoanalysis and psychotherapy as a vehicle for understanding masculinity. Perhaps the best known and leading exponents in this area were Freud and Jung, although others such as Fromm, Adler, Horney and Reik provided later accounts and additions to Freud's and Jung's work. Connell provides a detailed discussion of these theoretical works, but in essence they seek to align issues related to masculinity with the psyche. For example, Freud's articulation of the 'Oedipus Complex' (rivalry with the father and fear of castration), Jung's theorising of masculinity as a 'fear of the feminine', and Adler's proposition that the polarity of masculinity and femininity was based on the association of femininity with weakness. In general, the most important outcome of the psychoanalytic approach was the articulation of the heuristic nature of the unconscious. Horrocks (1994:19–20) argues that the articulation of the unconscious has enabled 'us to explain so much apparently bizarre behaviour...[because]...the unconscious utilizes contradictions, irrational juxtapositions, blends of images, projections and internalizations in a way that seems quite foreign to rational behaviour but often underlies it.'

The second major project Connell identified grew out of the development of social psychology, particularly the popular idea of 'sex role'. The perceived failure of 'naturalistic biologisim' and, in some areas, the psychoanalytic approach to 'account' for gender differences gave way to sex role attribution as the theoretical/explanatory means by which gender differences were created and sustained. The notion of sex role is, according to Connell (1995:22), the enactment of a set of expectations which are attached to one's sex and in any culture there are two quite distinct sex roles: a male one and a female one. The work of a number of writers (Hartley 1959, Kohlburg 1966, Gagnon & Simon 1973, Heilbrun 1976), support the notion that human behaviour is largely acquired through experience and socialisation. To this extent, it is easy to relate masculinity and femininity as external manifestations of behavioural expectations, which are the products of socialisation. However, it seems that the more the nature/nurture debate is investigated, the less clear we become about the relationship between nature and environment; furthermore, the debate does help us explore ways in which the lived experience of embodiment differs between men and women — if it differs at all on some things.

The third major project that Connell articulates concerns recent developments in anthropology, history and sociology. This project, which is discussed in more detail in the following section, has seen the rejection of the notion of a positivist science of masculinity in favour of illustrating social practice, through historical representation and ethnographical accounts, as the source of knowledge of and about masculinity.

Hegemonic masculinity

The concept of hegemonic masculinity has been detailed by a number of writers. Connell (1983:30–31), claimed that the most striking facet of the construction of hegemonic masculinity is the length and complexity of the process. It is not a well defined process that can be identified and attached to early childhood, schooling or even the transition into post-school life. Rather, it is a process that spans, at the very least, twenty years or more and is founded on a complex set of relationships that includes life history and experiences in the different stages of growth and development. In addition, the complexity of the process is compounded because it is at this time that one's life experiences are being expanded, negated and transformed into new ones.

While it is reasonable to say that we are now more discerning in the views being projected about masculinity, overwhelming traditional or entrenched assumptions about maleness and masculinity (in the singular sense) still exist. Historically, discourses (and the assumptions embedded in them) surrounding masculinity have effectively served to create and sustain dominant or hegemonic masculinity; and they have been powerful means by which men defined themselves as males and experienced their worlds as gendered being. While the attention has been focused on men in their social roles, less attention has been directed at ways in which men relate to their bodies and embodied behaviour.

Hegemonic masculinity has come to represent both that form of masculinity that is observed as socially and politically correct and the expectations of what males should do and how they should behave. In other words hegemonic masculinity represents the socially constructed patriarchal rules that accompany male role(s) and it defines the boundaries by which maleness (and therefore masculinity) are judged and/or deemed to be acceptable. To this end, the discourse performs ideological work in that it links apparently innate elements rather than those that are socially constructed; it serves to arbitrarily forge associations, which have no necessary relationship(s), in order to work as the vehicle to support the process of social ordering (Kirk 1994:2).

This process of social ordering has resulted in a situation where young males are driven towards attaining and continually demonstrating some kind of masculine identity by extremely subtle but powerful social and psychological forces. In addition, the impetus continues for older males because they are pressured to maintain and continue to demonstrate their masculinity. To illustrate these pressures, Samuel Osherson used the work of Mark Twain who observed that at about twelve, boys begin imitating a man and they go on doing that for the rest of their lives until they stop imitating and feel a deep and confident sense of their own manhood (1986:iv).

More recently we have seen the traditional notion of hegemonic masculinity weakening and destabilising slowly which has, in part, emanated from the recognition that construction of masculinity in its hegemonic form does not actually advantage men. While it is well argued that hegemonic masculinity and patriarchy support men and give meaning to social and cultural practices as well as the production and maintenance of the power relations of men over women, there is a significant difference between what patriarchy purports and supports and its subsequent value to men.

The idea that patriarchy and hence hegemonic masculinity is of value to all men is limited and limiting. Hegemonic masculinity has more to do with how select groups of men create and sustain positions of power and how they subsequently legitimate and reproduce the social relationships that generate their dominance. Hegemonic masculinity, then, primarily

> refers to competitive, physically aggressive males, who expose themselves to injury and risk taking activities, are often prone to bouts of violence, express themselves bodily, and indulge in sexist, racist, homophobic commentaries and practices. This is not to say that all males fit neatly into such categories...but alternative definitions of masculinity are considered only in relation to the dominant definition (Bricknell 1994:6–7).

Such disembodied constructs of what it means to be male result in an elevated form of masculinity determined by the patriarchal ideal and which in fact may only be represented by the characteristics of a few men. Yet by these means men and masculinity in general are defined (Carrigan et al 1987:92).

Validation of masculinity: 'I am therefore I must act'

The construction and maintenance of hegemonic masculinity has also seen the construction and maintenance of various forms of validation. What is striking in the discussions is that validation of masculinity is essentially a physical, embodied experience that involves a bodily expression of one's maleness.

Hearn (1994) cites the work of Christine Heward (1988) who argued that validation of masculinity is primarily achieved through institutionalised practices such as occupation, income, social position, family, sport and leisure activities. Heward modelled her concept on the family as the basic social unit and primary source of institutionalised socialisation practices. It is through their sons that parents work to ensconce the family's social position. Raising sons is about masculinising, and masculinising is about having a suitable occupation, income, social position and physical presence. Being able to support a wife and children (of whom at least one is male) is a transparent expression of heterosexual masculinity which allows the male (and others who support this model) to replicate and reproduce the essential institutionalised socialisation practices.

While the institutionalised practices described by Heward are about masculinising they are also central to the processes that validate masculinity in the hegemonic form. Hantover (1978:184–184) suggests that because of the cultural construction of masculinity men have a need to seek out opportunities to perform normatively appropriate male behaviours. This need arises from the hidden assumption that masculinity is not affirmed once and for all simply by genetic composition, but that it must be continually affirmed through ongoing action(s) — a line of argument that is troubling for those who would argue that maleness and masculinity is biologically constructed.

143

Even though Hantover's work is almost twenty years old, there is a large corroborating and growing literature, particularly since the 1980s, that addresses the issue of sex-role stereotyping and reinforcement. Examples can be readily found in the literatures on single-sex and coeducational schools, occupational choice and the well-known Bem sex-role inventory. While it can be argued that many of these works operated on the 'fringe' of more recently acknowledged issues, they have contributed significantly to grounding contemporary thinking about the process involved in the validation of masculinity.

Many of the masculinising processes identified so far include the particular characteristics of a male (as an individual) such as independence, pride, inner-strength, competitiveness, success, self-control and physical strength or prowess. These masculinising characteristics are reinforced through the sex-typing of toys, play, games and organised sports and social activities as well as choice of subjects at school and occupations in later life. For example, toy guns, cars and trucks and sporting activities such as football and soccer. Many of the things that are sex-typed as appropriate male behaviours or which assist socialising processes that help define masculinity are associated with high morbidity and mortality, particularly in young men.

Such activities include clubs or groups such as Boy Scouts, Boys' Brigade and Army Cadets and so on. While these might be 'little boys'' toys and activities, the argument can be put that they are really miniature versions of 'big boys'' toys and activities. Whether these toys, games and activities are used in play or part of 'real life', they serve to masculinise and validate the continuance of one's masculinity through the appeasement of 'training' boys in the masculine virtues and for adult males, to be seen in the sphere of masculine validation. In this way boys and young adult males are encultured or socialised to support and validate their masculinity as an ongoing process; and older males are encultured to want to be seen as the facilitators of these processes.

That the types of sex-typed games and toys for boys are almost all associated in 'real' life with risky if not potentially fatal activities seems so obvious; and, this link is carried on into adult life. Many of us in later life, when we reflect on our childhood, are sometimes surprised that we actually survived into adulthood! In effect, becoming masculine is about learning to adapt to and embody risky ways of living and being, not only in relation to what activities are engaged in, but also in relation to dismissing as unimportant, or ignoring, potentially serious symptoms and risk factors because that would be un-manly.

What is striking about these validation processes is the centrality of war and weaponry (and ultimately violence) which symbolises the nexus between expressed and embodied maleness and masculinity. As men in both the United States and British armies put it 'I've got a rifle, I've got a gun; my rifle's for killing, my gun's for fun' (Cornwall & Lindisfarne 1994:21). Furthermore, the expression of maleness and male violence in the social (public) domain and embodied maleness in the individual (private) domain is potentially seamless. These validation processes have created and sustain a metonymic relationship in that they associate men and masculinity with images and instruments of power and control.

144

Whether these instruments are military hardware, sports cars, body appendages, the sporting hero, the 'Marlboro Man' (and more recently the 'Solo Man'), they reveal the commodity logic which typifies capitalist formations. As a result, masculine identities can be located in

> the possessions which can be acquired or lost. Such are the implications of the aphorism, 'clothes do make the man' or the Texas wisdom that 'a man is no better than his horse and a man without a horse is no man at all' (Cornwall & Lindisfarne 1994:21).

Male violence, homophobia, misogyny and compulsory heterosexuality

Some of the most consequential and disturbing attributes that have been labelled as 'masculine' include aggression, toughness, forcefulness, power, tenacity and invincibility. These encultured attributes support the continued validation of masculinity through violence, almost as if, by the very nature of the discourse or describing language, violence is condoned. The important issue here is that violence is learned, not just as means of defending charges of 'unmanly' behaviour but also because it is perceived to be an effective, appropriate and hence acceptable way for boys and men to behave (Thompson 1987:155). More particularly, actual or potential violence is one of the central mechanisms through which males maintain power and control.

In providing an account of his school life, David Jackson (1990:188–189) pointed out that violence, in all its many forms, became an accepted, almost invisible part of school life and that violence was central to the 'male culture of toughness' and the process of masculine identification. In addition, daily beatings and fights as well as psychological violence were institutionally naturalised and taken to be part of daily life. He went on to suggest that the ideologies surrounding masculinity buttressed the aggressive ways in which boys relate to each other and 'put a premium on toughness and force'. If a boy is called a 'sissy', a 'wimp', a 'fag', a 'poofter' and so on, it means that he is perceived as not being masculine or is 'unmanly'; and there is enormous pressure to defend the allegations (regardless of their truth!). In my own school life, there were times when I was compelled to defend such allegations and when I did so I was told I 'hit like a girl' so I lost out on both counts.

Recently, the problem of male violence has become the focus of attention as it relates to playground violence, the role of the media, particularly television programs and computer games. Kate Legge, reporting in *The Australian Magazine* (1995:21) pointed out that

> multi-media entertainment is classic 'goodies vs baddies' stuff with one concession to the politically correct modern world; it is non-sexist. Girls participate in the mortal combat but not as damsels in distress. We have deconstructed the feminine mystique but left masculinity largely intact. Jason, the Star Ranger [The Power Rangers], is a man of few words who uses his hands and feet. Another macho man in emotional shutdown.

145

A number of possible explanations about why violence is such an entrenched factor in masculinising processes have been proposed. Thompson suggests that violence is the tool which maintains the two most prominent socialising forces in a boy's life; homophobia and misogyny. Homophobia (the fear of gay men or those believed to be gay) as well as the fear of being labelled gay operates as a masculinising force in patriarchy because to be gay is to be stereotypically feminised. It is, then, a process which effectively differentiates a 'man's man' from a 'man who has sex with other men'; although the issue of bisexuality is a confounding problematic. Misogyny is linked, in this configuration, to homophobia (for men) in a complex arrangement of fear and dichotomous logic that defines maleness and non-femaleness. While these two forces (homophobia and misogyny) are targeted at different victims, they are, for the most part, aligned in that they are an expression of the hatred of feminine qualities. Therefore, if a boy is called a 'poofter' or a 'girl' he becomes potentially not only the victim of other boys' homophobia but also a victim of his own (Thompson 1987:156). To this extent, the notion of 'compulsory heterosexuality' potentially is as important in validating masculinity in patriarchy as it is for defining the roles and identities of women (see Rich 1980). Put simply (if that is possible in this context), men in a patriarchal society do not want to be like women or are fearful of being like them because women's oppression and subordination are central to male power, individually and collectively; and male power is maintained by violent means. So becoming male is heavily affected by fear of a whole range of other (mostly negative) forces that are ultimately embodied by individual men.

While violence is strongly related to homophobia and misogyny in the context in which Thompson presents it, violence is a dominant feature of male lives. Cornwall and Lindisfarne (1994:15) suggest that resorting to violence can be interpreted as potency, strength and machismo. Equally, however, it can be interpreted as a brute ignorance or a pathetic fragility. Interpretations of violence such as domestic beatings, racist attacks, child abuse or poofter-bashing depend on perceptions of legitimacy and provocation. While some people might applaud a violent response that others deplore, an individual's reactions are not necessarily constant. At different stages in the process of negotiating masculinities, and according to the different perspectives of the actors and their audiences, attributes of masculinity can and do change rapidly. This idea is supported by McElhinny (1994) who described the relation between force and emotion as contingent. Resorting to violence, which is often physical, in some circumstances may well be seen as the 'manly thing to do' while refusing to be violent may be seen to be 'wimpish' (even though it may be a demonstration of self-control and reason). To engage in a fight and lose might also be more demoralising than refusing to be involved in the first place. As a result, the emotional catalyst for violence is very much tied to the social and psychological forces which lead males to want and need to be seen as masculine.

The acts involved in validation of one's masculinity are inherently linked to the physical body and its size, shape, strength, perceived invincibility and subsequent performance, whether publicly or privately (through sexual activity and reproduction).

146

Male embodiment and experienced masculinity

Within the framework of studies on masculinity, the body has maintained a central position. The centrality of physical difference has been used as a means of contextualising and in some instances attempting to justify the existence of gender difference. From the point of view of psychoanalysis, this centrality rests with the protection of the body from castration and feminising; and from the social psychology perspective it rests with the physical enactment of ascribed roles. From a biological perspective, the genetic structure and hormonal balance of the body is the primary focus. At some points in a man's life these various influences come together, and at other times they are points of tension.

Embodiment has become a main feature in much of the modern discourse about gendered social life. This field has been led predominantly by women researching and writing in the area of female embodiment. Lawler (1991:66) argued that the importance of the body in social life has been overlooked in favour of what Turner (1984) called 'sociological determinism'. As a result of this determinism, the body has largely been excluded from sociological investigation because sociology has been primarily concerned with the dichotomy of self and society rather than the issue of nature and culture. There has been little attention paid to male embodied experience, in contrast to the voluminous literature concerning women, women's bodies and embodied experiences. Simone de Beauvoir's *The Second Sex* (1953), for example, is theoretically and philosophically based and primarily focused on female experience, including embodiment.

While Beauvoir's work has been central to feminist studies, there is no male equivalent of this text. What work has been done by male existentialist philosophers, such as Merleau-Ponty, Sartre and Heidegger, has addressed the issue of embodiment (and embodied knowing) as an intellectual or consciousness-related activity, conducted from a social organisation or group level, with little or no concern for the individual's sense of embodiment as a social being who also inhabits a physical body. In other words, the question of what it is like to live in a male body has not been asked. The bigger question, 'what is it to be?' has seemed to be the most self-evident. Except for Beauvoir, this has not been a gendered question.

How is a body experienced as a healthy entity and how does it relate to the experience of illness, disability and disease? This further emphasises our lack of knowledge about embodied masculinity, the lived experience of being male and how (and to what extent) these experiences impact on men individually and collectively. As Turner (1984:49) argued, the body is both natural and cultural and we cannot deny the corporeality of human existence and consciousness.

Connell (1983, 1987, 1995) has placed great emphasis on the centrality of the body to issues surrounding masculinity and has argued that concern for the body (in the lived sense) has been neglected in the debates on and about masculinity. He contended that

[t]he surface on which cultural meanings are ascribed is not featureless, and it does not stay still...[b]odies in their own rights as bodies, do matter. They age, get sick, enjoy, engender, give birth. There is an irreducible bodily dimension in experience and practice...One of the few compelling things the male role literature and books about men did was to catalogue problems with male bodies (1995:51).

In a recent review of Connell's *Masculinities*, McLean (1995) challenges Connell because his project on masculinity both represents and reflects the dominant patriarchal system that Connell critiques, yet that same system supports his work. McLean notes that Connell's personal involvement in his work, and the dilemmas it raises for him personally as a man, are curiously missing from his texts.

The way in which the male body is socially constructed — as a social and physical entity — is also integral to the examination of the notion of embodiment and masculinity. Women's bodies are culturally constructed as open: open to conception and birth, menses and penetration (usually by a penis). By virtue of their openness, women's bodies are also constructed as vulnerable and incomplete which makes them weak and a target for conquest (usually by men). Much of the pornographic literature exemplifies this vulnerability and openness simply by the posturing or posing that is used. Men's bodies, on the other hand, are constructed as closed and hence more complete, strong and invincible (Buchbinder 1994:42). More generally, the ideal types of masculinity, as they are socially expressed, mimic these ideal physical types. The construction of men's bodies in this way is perhaps best exemplified by the difficulty some men have with the concept of anal sex and in particular anal sex in male-male sexual activity.

The completeness, strength and invincibility of the male body is also encoded in our views about the ideal male physique. We have entered a social period where 'working out' and body building are becoming increasingly common. While the female body conventionally has an image of softness and attractiveness, men's bodies conventionally have a presence dependent on the promise of or the actual power they 'embody' (Connell 1983:18). The ideal form then has become one of sharp definition, hardness, strength, a body that exudes 'masculine presence'. By contrast, the less than ideal male form is represented by the 'five stone weakling' who constantly has sand kicked in his face at the beach!

It would seem that there are two critical areas of the male body: the head (the source of intellectual and organisational power), and the penis. According to Horrocks (1994:162), the penis is the source of men's greatest feeling of power and likewise the source of the greatest feelings of weakness as well as the source of men's expression of love, hate, fear, tenderness, contempt, friendship and disgust as well as the place from which no emotions can be shown at all. A man's feeling towards his penis is sometimes a reflection of how he feels about himself: proud, shy, afraid, loving angry and ignorant. What Horrocks is suggesting may well appear to be contradictory in that it focuses on expression of a man's emotional state, yet in the descriptive semantics surrounding maleness and masculinity emotions do not rate highly or overtly. Herein lies the confusion inherent in male embodiment.

As discussed earlier, the work of Cornwall and Lindisfarne (1994) and McElhinny (1994) on male violence upholds the notion that the penis is central to the expression of a man's emotion across the spectrum of emotions ranging from hate and contempt to love and tenderness and in particular frustration and fear. In support, the more recent debate on what induces men to rape and indulge in other violent acts is couched in the view that it is one way that men can gain control or dominate their emotions when no other avenue is open to them. While this might seem an unacceptable reason for explaining these acts, the intent is not to provide justification but to highlight the lack of investigation in this area. Further, the representation of the penis is central to the significance of the organ. It is referred to as 'the weapon', 'the python', 'the rhythm stick' and 'the tool', all of which support the constructed dominance of the male and the symbolism of the male body as complete, self-sufficient, potent and above all strong, invincible and hard with the ability to control (by penetration).

The penis is also central to performance outside that related to sexual activity. Consider the phrase 'keep your pecker up' when someone is depressed or upset. In relation to sexual activity, however, the penis performs amazing work because it is perceived as a panacea for many female problems. For example, in a male environment, it is common to hear that a woman's temperament could be improved with a 'good lay'. Eva Figes (1978:23) used the experience of Simone de Beauvoir who, in her autobiography, recorded that when her work, *The Second Sex*, was published in France, some of the vituperation heaped upon her were many suggestions that 'what was really wrong with her was that she had never been "properly" fucked'.

Embodied masculinity, the emotionless man and men's health

The power of the penis is particularly problematic as it relates to the expression of the gamut of emotions experienced by men. For men to be seen to express emotion(s) in other than socially acceptable ways is to risk being called a 'wimp', a 'sissy', a 'poofter' and above all less than the 'ideal (hegemonic) man'. This is certainly evidenced by the difficulty some men (and women) have with the concept of the sensitive new age guy (SNAG). According to Buchbinder (1994:18–19) this politically correct (from the feminist point of view) new age man is supposedly more sensitive to women's personal and political needs, more self-aware and more respectful of the earth and nature than his peers who rape and pillage. Unfortunately, some women and men alike view this new age man warily. Buchbinder continues:

> For women, the question is, can the leopard change its spots? Or, to employ another cliche, is New Age Man really the same old wolf decked out in new sheep's clothing? Is his new-found sensitivity and so on merely a strategy to keep things as they are, allowing him to continue to prey sexually on women? For some men, on the other hand, New Age Man may appear to

149

be a wimp, a man who has sold to women his birthright as a male (Buchbinder 1994:19).

It is not surprising that we have, particularly in Australia with its strongly entrenched masculine cultural identity, a situation where men are reticent about expressing their feelings, fears and uncertainties, except when they are expressed violently, and in some instances, towards themselves. Stephen Firn (1995:60) from his research and work in conducting sexuality workshops, reported that the men express their dislike about feeling compelled to be always seen to be coping and in control regardless of how they really feel. Further, they rarely, if ever, reveal their emotions because it suggests weakness and failure in their personal and professional lives.

For men, who have embodied traditional notions of masculinity, expressing emotions is to be 'soft' and it is to this 'soft man' that criticism is levelled because he has given in to feminism and hence lost his 'masculinity'. Men are indoctrinated to be outwardly unemotional and rational; Horrocks (1994:107) described this as 'male autism' whereby men are in a state of being cut off from their feelings, expressiveness and contact with others. He went on to point out that male autism can be understood in the context of Sartre's analysis of 'bad faith' which is the condition of being something that one is fundamentally not. As Sartre suggested, the public does not want a grocer who dreams, they demand that he limit himself to his function as a grocer (in Horrocks 1994:109).

It is becoming increasingly obvious that the emotional costs associated with masculinity are immense and far reaching. In attempting to validate masculinity and masculine identity along hegemonic lines, men are in fact emotionally crippled because:

> [m]anhood as we know it in our society requires such a self-destructive identify, a deep masochistic self-denial, a shrinkage of the self, a turning away from whole areas of life, that a man who obeys the demands of masculinity has become only half-human... . This is the cryptic message of [hegemonic] masculinity: don't accept who you are. Conceal your weaknesses, your tears, your fear of death, your love for others. Conceal your impotence. Conceal your potency. Disparage women, since they remind you too much of your own feminine side. Disparage gay men since that's too close to the bone as well. Fake your behaviour. Dominate others, then you can fool everyone, especially yourself, that you feel powerful (Horrocks 1994:25).

Summary and conclusion

The push for and subsequent establishment of the women's health agenda originated out of issues surrounding the medicalisation of women's health (and their ill-health) and the patriarchal nature of the health care system. The health system as it was constructed did not meet the health needs of women and, in fact, promoted medical intervention in otherwise 'normal' women's bodily functions and processes. Only recently have we witnessed the emergence of concern over the issues related to men's health but this movement is driven by rather different forces. As patriarchy does not serve to advantage all men, neither does a patriarchal health system meet the health needs of all men. Rather, we have a system that is based on an illness model, technology and an intricate set of power relations that are manifested in the micro and macro levels in the organisation of health services.

The obstacles and problems that are created for men in attempting to uphold or fulfil the social rules that have been constructed for the masculine role are problematic for men's physical, social and psychological well-being and these problems have been recognised and articulated in the more recent drive for the establishment of a men's health agenda. The basis for this agenda has been the recognition of the impact of increasing levels of unemployment and economic downturn shown in higher rates of suicide and mental ill-health among men, the startling difference in mortality and morbidity rates between males and females, as well as a higher incidence of work related accidents and health risks among men. As Richard Fletcher pointed out, the most publicly available data were the Australian Bureau of Statistics compilation of mortality rates for males and females in Australia. As a result of his investigation he was surprised to find that males were dying at greater rates in all age groups, sometimes by a ratio of 2:1. But he was even more surprised to find that no-one in the health services or beyond that saw these figures as a problem (cited by Ots 1994:2).

The men's health agenda has also extended to take into account the health related issues that accompany masculinities and in particular the validation processes that construct masculinity. Questions are being asked: why do men more readily engage in high risk leisure activities?; why do some men in high risk occupations disregard occupational health and safety precautions?; why is violent or aggressive behaviour an acknowledged, and in some contexts an accepted, masculine trait?; why do men repress their emotional and 'feminine' side in favour of a 'real tough son of a bitch' identity?; and, what are the outcomes for the continuation of this form of masculine identity and expression?

Answers lie somewhere in the construction and maintenance of masculinity in the hegemonic form, in establishing how pervasive it is, and by what means these issues can be addressed as mainstream issues in western patriarchal culture.

NOTES

1 Sociolinguistics is concerned with how language is used in its social context and how its form and function changes across different cultures and social situations within one culture. Sociolinguistics relies on analysis of how people talk to each other in everyday settings, how talk is organised, what makes it understandable and how it is interpreted (Stubbs 1983:7, 44).

2 Semiotics is the study of systems of signs or symbols that are produced, recognised and used by different cultures at given points in time. The signs or symbols are not concrete but fluid and are redefined and reorganised according to that cultures transition/development, change or reorientation. These recognised signs and symbols are powerful influences over how we think and function as a society and personally.

151

REFERENCES

Bricknell L 1994 Designer males: masculinity, sexuality, personal relations and the quest for identity. Proceedings of Men's health and family preservation conference, Ausmed, Melbourne

Brod H 1987 The new men's studies: From feminist theory to gender scholarship. Hypatia 2(1):184

Buchbinder D 1994 Masculinities and identities. Melbourne University Press, Melbourne

Carrigan T, Connell B, Lee J 1987 Towards a new sociology of masculinity. In: Brod H (ed) The making of masculinities: the new men's studies. Allen & Unwin, Boston

Connell R W 1983 Which way is up? Essays in class, sex and culture. George Allen & Unwin, Sydney

Connell R W 1987 Gender and power. Allen & Unwin, Sydney

Connell R W 1995 Masculinities. Allen & Unwin, Sydney

Cornwall A, Lindisfarne N 1994 Dislocating masculinities: gender, power and anthropology. In: Cornwall A, Lindisfarne N (eds) Dislocating masculinity. Routledge, London

de Beauvoir S 1953 The second sex. Translated by H M Parshley. Penguin, Harmondsworth

Figes E 1978 Patriarchal attitudes. Virago, London

Firn S 1995 Peril of the stiff upper lip. Nursing Times 91(25):60

Friend R A 1987 Sexual identity and human diversity: Implications for nursing practice. Holistic Nursing Practice 1(4):21–41

Gagnon J, Simon W 1973 Sexual conduct: the social sources of sexuality. Aldine, Chicago

Hantover J 1978 The boy scouts as validation of masculinity. Journal of Social Issues 34(1):184–195

Hartley R E 1959 Sex role pressures and the socialisation of the male child. Psychological Reports 5:457–468

Hearn J 1994 Research in men and masculinities: some sociological issues and possibilities. Australian and New Zealand Journal of Sociology 30(1):47–70

Heilbrun A B 1976 Measurement of masculine and feminine sex-role identities as independent dimensions. Journal of Consulting and Clinical Psychology 44:183–190

Horrocks R 1994 Masculinity in Crisis. St. Martin's Press, New York

Jackson D 1990 Unmasking masculinity: a critical autobiography. Unwin Hymen, London

Kimmel M 1987 Changing men: new directions in research on men and masculinity. Sage, Thousand Oaks

Kirk D 1994 School physical education, embodied masculinity and health. Proceedings of Men's health and family preservation conference. Ausmed, Melbourne

Kohlburg L A A 1966 A cognitive developmental analysis of children's sex-role concepts and attitudes. In: Maccoby E (ed) The development of sex-differences. Stanford University Press, Stanford

Lawler J 1991 Behind the screens: nursing, somology and the problem of the body. Churchill Livingstone, Melbourne

Legge K 1995 Some mother's do have 'em. The Australian Magazine (March 11–12):21–29

McElhinny B 1994 An economy of effect: objectivity, masculinity and the gendering of police work. In Cornwall A and Lindisfarne N (eds) Dislocating masculinity. Routledge, London

McLean C 1995 Review of R W Connell, Masculinities. Australian Feminist Studies (22):168–169

Morgan D 1992 Discovering men. Routledge, London

Osherson S 1986 Finding our father: the unfinished business of manhood. Free Press, London

Ots J 1994 The social meaning of health and men. Proceedings of Men's health and family preservation conference, Ausmed, Melbourne

Pleck J H 1987 The theory of male sex-role identity: its rise and fall, 1936 to the present. In: Brod H (ed) The making of masculinities: the new men's studies. Allen & Unwin, Boston

Rich A 1980 Compulsory heterosexuality. Journal of Women in Culture and Society 5(4)631–660

Rubin G 1975 The traffic in women: notes on the 'political economy' of sex. In: Reiter R R (ed) Towards an anthropology of women. Monthly Review Press, New York

Stubbs M 1983 Discourse analysis: the sociolinguistic analysis of natural language. Blackwell, Oxford

Thompson C 1987 A new vision of masculinity. In: Abbott F (ed) New men, new minds: breaking male tradition. Crossing Press, Freedom

Turner BS 1984 The body and society: explorations in social theory. Basil Blackwell, Oxford

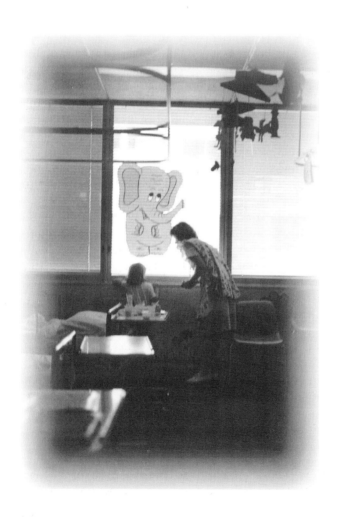

10

Embodied self, human biology and experience

Maureen Boughton

Introduction

In this chapter I intend to examine ways in which concepts of self are intrinsically embodied and, in relation to some experiences, biologically determined. The role of one's personal and socially constructed sense of the body will be examined in relation to forming concepts of self and identity. The concept of self as it is affected by the biological body will be explored using menopause, ageing and chronic illness as examples.

There has been little interest in the body in nursing until recently and Morgan and Scott (1993:1) argue that this is also true for sociology. They suggest that, to a large extent, this is because much research is located within universities and other institutions which have been traditionally (and many remain so) associated with 'cultivation of the mind and with the deployment of reason'. The shift in interest and focus on the body in sociology, along with the movement of nurse education from hospitals to tertiary institutions, has probably been partly responsible for generating nursing research on the body. Traditionally, there has been a preoccupation with research and teaching that is of a scientific nature, particularly in health care; consequently, topics such as the lived body have been largely ignored. More recently, nurses have recognised that their 'doing business' with patients frequently involves the body as it is lived and in providing bodily care — an area which Lawler's (1991) study addressed.

The concept of holistic care, in which all aspects of the person can be addressed, has been espoused for more than two decades in nursing. The claim that nurses care for the whole person is an attempt to show that we acknowledge the person's cultural, psychosocial, sexual, environmental and physical individuality. The fact that nursing adopted the medical model, with its inherent ideas of the body and mind as separate, has been problematic for nursing, hindering any comprehensive and unconditional adoption of this concept. Therefore, the formal, mainstream emphasis in nursing care, despite the rhetoric of holism, has remained on care of the physical body and not necessarily the person as an embodied being.

The body is the mediator between people's self-identity and, like many, Turner (1992:18) and Grosz (1994:27) contend that the body is bound into society and regulated by history and culture, in particular. Human embodiment is affected by interactions between the body (as a physical entity), society, history and culture; social meanings associated with the body become internalised in the context of culture, exerting a powerful influence on an individual's sense of self.

Influences of history on the formation of concepts of self and identity

The question, 'what is the body?', has been asked, debated, pondered and philosophised for centuries. The *Australian Oxford Dictionary* (1986) defines body as 'material frame of man [sic] or animal'. This conception of the body as a thing, with a given status, unchangeable, passive and inert is reflective of the natural sciences. As a physical thing, the body is presumed to be fundamentally biological and immune from cultural, social and historical factors. However, Synnott (1993:7) says that, historically, opinions have differed dramatically; and to illustrate, he provides these quotations from famous philosophers.

—The body is the tomb of the soul (Plato).

—Your body is the temple of the Holy Spirit (Saint Paul).

—The human body may be considered as a machine (Descartes).

—The body is what I immediately am...I am my body (Sartre).

Each of these concepts of the body reflects its location in relation to particular philosophies and world views, which change over time as the body differs in its significance both in a physical and social sense.

Synnott (1993:37) argues that any construction of the body is a construction of the self as embodied, which ultimately influences how our bodies are treated and how we live our lives. Drawing on his work, I will explore the principal themes or influences that historically have influenced thinking about the body, embodiment and the formation of self and identity.

Early philosophers

The Greek philosophers could not come to any consensus about the body. The Greeks glorified the body and their culture was body-centred, but no particular theory prevailed. There were, however, two opposing schools of thought, the first of which arose from the Cyrenaic school founded by Aristippus (c.435–366BC), a friend of Socrates. Aristippus claimed that 'bodily pleasures are far better than mental pleasures' (Laertius 1972 cited in Synnott 1993). The second and diametrically opposing view was held by the Epicureans. Epicurus (341–270 BC) believed that whilst the body is good, the mind is better — early evidence of the separation of mind and body and superiority of mind over body — a theme that later become known as Cartesian dualism (after Descartes).

Religious influences

The fourth century BC witnessed the emergence of a most unpopular philosophy affecting the body directly — the period when abstinence was the key feature in an attempt to cultivate a divine nature. The philosophy was founded by Orpheus and at this time the body was regarded as the tomb of the soul. Socrates and Plato both saw the body (*soma*) as the tomb (*sema*) of the soul describing the body as a hindrance enslaving and shackling the superior soul. The body was thought to be evil and the soul only liberated at the time of death (a body/soul dualism). Plato, however, was somewhat of a contradiction in his thoughts on the body in that he also associated a beautiful body with an advancement along the path to 'Absolute Beauty and God'. So according to Plato, the body was capable of both leading to or away from God.

Aristotle (384–322 BC), who had been Plato's student, rejected the body/ soul dualism. He dismissed the question of whether body and soul are one as an unnecessary problem, although he held the view that the soul was superior to the body — evidence again of attempts to construct some parts of being as superior to other, more physical parts. Aristotle elevated the mind even further, by proposing that the intellect *was* man (sic). The body was not seen as negative; rather, it was not as significant as the intellect.

In its early years, Christian thought was strongly influenced by Stoicism, which was the dominant philosophy at the turn of the millennium in the Roman Empire. While the early Christians dabbled with several different paradigms of the body, there remained a tension and ambiguity between the body as both a positive and negative entity. They viewed the body as consisting of three components — the physical, the spiritual and the mystical. Synnott (1993:12–14) provides examples from biblical writings to demonstrate that within the teachings of Christ, caring for the physical body figured prominently. Saint Paul, for example, described the body as a temple of the Holy Spirit, which contrasts starkly with the earlier view of Orpheus that the body was a tomb.

In the early centuries of the Christian Church, there was a high priority given to asceticism, a dedication of the self to God expressed in martyrdom, virginity and celibacy. A dualistic arrangement of body and soul was widely accepted and even though both were considered beautiful in their own right, the beauty of the body compared with the soul was relatively unimportant. There is also evidence of an ongoing dilemma where, at times, the physical body was encountered with enthusiasm, albeit in a context that arranged the body as inferior to the soul.

157

The body enjoyed something of a resurgence during the Renaissance in the fourteenth century. Italian artists presented the body as something beautiful in paint and sculpture, emphasising the body as a thing of beauty to be appreciated for its own, purely secular sake. This period witnessed the change from the ascetic idea of the body to a view that the body was beautiful, good, personal and private; however, ascetic ideas were not displaced totally.

During this time, silencing of public discourse about sexual matters and 'private parts' of the body began, as did an ideologically driven move to distance self and bodily functions from the body itself (Synnott 1993:18–20). This silence still has an influence on current thinking in relation to the body and various events that affect it, for example menopause. The various reasons why such a move should occur is debated, but Elias' (1985) work on the civilizing process has been influential.

Cartesian influences

Western philosophy has maintained a dualist view of varying forms about the body; however, the influence of Descartes' thinking has been the most profound. And despite his acknowledgment of the interdependence of the body and the mind, he is usually attributed as having originated Cartesian dualism, that is, the conceptual split between the mind and the body. As Lawler (1991:55) pointed out, Descartes, in his Sixth Meditation (1986:159) wrote

> I am not only lodged in my body like a pilot in his ship, but besides that I am joined to it very closely and indeed so compounded and intermingled with my body, that I form, as it were, a single whole with it.

What Descartes actually accomplished is not only a mind-body separation but the separation of soul from nature. Grosz (1994:6–7) points out that he 'distinguished two kinds of substances: a thinking substance (*res cogitans*, mind) from an extended substance (*res extensa*, body)'. He considered the body to be part of nature but not the mind; consciousness is placed outside of the world so that it becomes 'an island unto itself'. It is positioned outside of the body and nature as well as being removed from any 'direct contact with other minds as a socio-cultural community'.

Development of the postmodern body

Dualistic constructs have pervaded philosophical thought for centuries in spite of (or possibly because of) its posing irresolvable philosophical problems. The assumption that body and mind are distinct entities, mutually exclusive, and exhaustive, inhabiting there own self-contained precinct is problematic. The nexus between mind and body that results with reductionism denies or explicitly stands outside any interaction between mind and body. It has led to perennial, prolific investigations and writings about the body as object or subject and the body and self; often this has emphasised (apparent) differences rather than interconnections.

As a consequence of seventeenth century Cartesianism, the body is primarily regarded as an object for the natural sciences. The notion of 'the person as an assemblage of traits or variables such as anxiety, control and self-esteem, which are viewed as context-free elements to be combined according to formal laws that can be discovered through the scientific method' flows from the implicit acceptance of Cartesian notions of the self (Leonard 1989:41). The self is viewed as subject possessing a body and existing in the object, that is, the world of environment.

According to Turner (1992:31), there has been a major shift in both the social sciences and humanities during the 1980s towards exploration of the problem of the body in social life. Prior to this period, the area of human embodiment has been neglected largely because of the implicit acceptance of the Cartesian tradition of dealing with the mind and body separately. In that tradition, the human body is 'merely a machine driven by mechanical causality and susceptible to mathematical analysis' (Leder 1984:29–30).

The notion that the body is like a machine has served to advance modern medicine and create possibilities for treating specific organ systems both medically and surgically, but the resultant isolation of self from body in this framework is inevitable. Indeed, medicine as a science seems to demand a mind/body split in order to establish a discourse of the body-as-a-machine. Such objectification of the body repudiates the somatically felt and tactile-kinaesthetic body that is the experience of the person who inhabits this body-as-machine. Marcel (cited by Zaner 1964:21) accuses natural scientific inquiry of dissolving the lived unity of experience. He theorises that I and my body are unified and that consciousness is embodied by the specific individual. He argues that who I am is crucially dependent upon my having a specific body, which I do not (and can not) share with any other individual. The body as it is experienced and the object body of science is one and the same because there is no distinction between subject and object at the level of individual human embodiment, no detachment and no within/without; rather, we are embodied beings.

Developing a sense of an embodied self

The concept of self and the way in which we experience ourselves as embodied can be understood as located simultaneously in three dimensions — biologically, historically and culturally. Sheets-Johnstone (1992:3) refers to cultural seduction when she contends that we no longer have a 'living sense of ourselves'. This aspect of ourselves seems to have vanished in the wake of the dominant body view held by society. On a daily basis we are exposed to information, some of which arises from modern science and technology, about what we should and shouldn't be putting into our mouths, how we can get more enjoyment out of our sexual relationships, how to manage our stress and what stress can do to the physical body and how to go about creating a more perfect body. We are bombarded with what Sheets-Johnstone calls 'popular body noise' (p.3).

To greater and lesser degrees, the information about who we should be as embodied characters is internalised so that individual identities are moulded and shaped by the immediate environment. Individual responses to situations are often suppressed in favour of a more culturally accepted view. Attitudes and values are seen to be ingrained. Bordo (1991:119–121) gives an example of a study that demonstrates how some black children embody white values. When the children were asked to answer a series of questions about two dolls — one black and one white — all the positive characteristics were attributed to the white doll and the negative characteristics to the black doll. The children had developed their beliefs about self-identity based on the white Anglo-Saxon image; and they were embarrassed to say they were like the black doll. Being asked to face the reality of acknowledging their black colouring served as a reinforcement of feelings of inadequacy and inferiority. It reminded them of their 'place' in the world. The difference creates an imbalance of power, rendering those deemed to be different or in the minority, disempowered. Skin colouring is initially simply biologically determined; however, before a child is old enough to make any sense of their world they are exposed to cultural ideals and stereotypical images of what is desirable in the physical body — and by default, what can be internalised as desirable in the (embodied) person.

The body is simultaneously biological and social. The body is a biological organism inextricably linked to social processes and culture. A newborn baby starts its life (usually) as a boy or girl with a species-specific nervous system connected to a brain, organs and muscles. The baby grows and develops in a social world and becomes a distinct entity in the world in which he or she lives, set apart from others by corporeal skills, habits and particular styles of expression. It is the individual person's unique way of being-in-the-world. The body is not only defined by social relations but it can also be used to define the social relations and to integrate a community. The child is able to do this in two ways:

1 a universal body experience that is the common body; and
2 the particular body experience.

It is this second way of experiencing the body that accounts for differences in gender, ethnicity, age and family. Carkeek and James (1992:73–76) argue that we express, by way of symbols, socially constructed practices, which can gain the power to structure and over-determine processes of social formation. The symbols are created by people and it is precisely these symbols that then 'define society, social behaviour and relationships and even their sense of body, from which the symbols derived' (p.74). An elaborate code can be formed from bodily symbols, which regulate dress, posture, etiquette, social contact, expressions of respect and a range of other social behaviours. Alone, the consequences are curbed but as a generalised code they define and affirm social order.

The body and self-identity are integrally related with our upbringing having a major effect on the way we develop our self-identity. Gender roles are differentiated in the way girls and boys are expected to walk, talk and dress and which helps to identify their masculinity or femininity; these roles are derived from 'given' biological, physical differences that define one form as male and the other as female. This occurs prior to the child's ability to recognise himself or herself as biologically male or female, assuming an acceptance that there is an anatomical difference between females and males.

However, Scott and Morgan (1993:5–6) argue that this view is problematic and that it is based on an ideological assumption that becomes more fragile when it is considered in its historical context. They say that there is evidence to suggest that, prior to the eighteenth century (and some claim even until the beginning of the nineteenth century), males and females were thought to have basically the same genitalia except that the female's were located inside the body rather than outside as were the male's.

Hermaphrodites and transsexuals present other kinds of troubling issues for those who argue that the sociably enacted self is based on a particular biologically given (and driven) base. These minority groups are generally dealt with by placing them outside the socially defined boundaries of gender categories. In Australia (and many other countries), by law, you remain male or female according to the sex you were determined to be at birth. This means that, in the case of transsexuals and some hermaphrodites, self-identity as it is embodied may be expressed as opposite to the biologically ascribed sexual identity.

Identity and biologically defined sexed being is a complex issue in which social forces play a large role. For example, Reiger (1987:105) in her discussion of Elshtain's (1984) and Kovel's (1983) propositions regarding embodiment and identity formation, highlights the fact that a child's sense of self is formed out of an 'embodied engagement with the world'. The child actively takes in their world to become part of self and in the process they will inevitably encounter sexed bodies.

Bordo (1990:109) asserts also that 'no body can escape either the imprint of culture or its gendered meanings'. Gender differences are reinforced throughout life but the absolute differences between the sexes is exaggerated and similarities disregarded. Both the social and biological sciences began to highlight obsessively the differences between female and male sexuality, social roles and economic spheres as attempts to explain sexual division in patriarchal societies. Less attention, in all manner of disciplines, has been paid to similarities between male and female sexualised, socialised, and embodied being.

The body, self and identity

Game (1991:192) purports that truth is found in the body. She argues that 'the body provides the basis for a different conception of knowledge: we know with our bodies'. The body is not just a skeleton with organs, flesh and skin, it is primarily the means through which we develop a sense of self and come to know the world. Bodies and body parts are steeped in cultural symbolism, which can be both private and public, positive and negative, political, economic, sexual, moral and very often controversial. Synnott (1993:1) describes the body as being 'sponge-like' in its ability to absorb meanings. At every age, different meanings are imposed within both social and political categories. The body, in Turner's view (1992:17), is 'simultaneously, conjointly and concurrently socially constructed and organically founded'.

Attributes of the body such as age, gender, and colour have a significant role in our social identities and are principal determinants of our lives. The way we appear physically to ourselves and others is based, in part, on a judgement of our bodily attributes. For example, we may be seen in varying degrees of attractiveness, deemed to be short(er) or tall(er), fat(ter) or thin(ner) or to be afflicted with a physical handicap. Social responses to these and other attributes affect the way we see ourselves and they also may affect our life chances.

Turner (1992:37) argues that to talk about one's identity is difficult without making reference to a specific body. We can have memories and social records in diaries but being a specific person requires a specific body — one we recognise as belonging to ourselves in a unique way. Embodiment also has crucial implications for some health related issues such as menopause, acquired disability, infertility, chronic illness and ageing as well our attitudes to a variety of health related behaviours.

Synnott (1993:2) asserts that, in this period in history, we probably think and worry about our body all the time and more than any other thing. There is an acute emphasis on AIDS, beauty, death, face and fat, hair, weight, sex and pimples. There is a centredness (almost to the point of fixation on the body) in spite of 'historically privileged mind over matter'.

The body, self and age(ing)

The degree of significance and the concentration of our somatic concerns change as we age. Around puberty the individual is concerned with bodily changes because these essentially change identity at a time when one's sense of self is still being shaped in a relatively active way. But our identities continue to shift as we experience alterations to the way our bodies look, feel, and work — or don't work, as the case may be.

Menstruation is privileged as a significant biological change bought about by hormonal activity and which marks a shift in definitions of self from the premenstrual to fertile and reproductive possibilities; in the biological sense, one enters one's sexually 'mature' years. Menopause, the cessation of menstruation, marks yet another shift in definition of self. While hormonal changes are responsible for the transition from a reproductive stage into a post-reproductive stage (as they are at menstruation), menopause is defined medically as a disease.

The social stereotype of the middle-aged or ageing person is hardly an enviable one. The focus moves from the person with a purpose who is valuable contributor to society to one where the same person may be seen as a drain on government funds. They may be regarded as less employable or unemployable, have a greater need for medical care and become reliant upon welfare services for a basic existence. The individual's self-identity involves change over time and we transit from altered relationships between the body, self, self image and lifestyle. In ageing, changes are not episodic as they are in illness; rather, they are thematic and progressive. The biological body becomes less active, its shape changes, faces become etched with lines, eyesight deteriorates, hearing becomes less acute, bones become brittle and flesh begins to sag. This body may be viewed as not only object but as an obstacle of the self. Gadow (1980:178) says in this instance the self will endeavour to overcome limitations, not only by extending given capabilities but cultivating new ones.

The negative view of the body comes from the way in which the body is actively hostile to a person's intentions and wishes as an embodied person. The ageing body can be felt as an oppressor demeaning and humiliating the self; progressively, the body refuses to perform basic functions reliably producing a disengagement between body and self. The body behaves in an unfamiliar way as it ages, and this can be experienced as conspicuous, negative, and typifying the worst of commonly portrayed images of ageing. Ageing people may regret the loss of their familiar body as their hair greys and other realities of ageing appear such as wrinkling skin and curved posture. The previously familiar body takes on a certain strangeness and in our present western society this is emphasised by the knowledge that judgements are based on the physical body as seen by the other.

Because aesthetic regard toward the body is pronounced in our society, an ageing body can become the focus of attention and may engage our full concentration. It may not matter how much the person may feel the same with the same needs and desires, they are faced with others' changed perceptions of their role and function(s) within society. The stereotype of an older person may make it difficult for individuals to develop a livable relationship with their changing body.

The mature female: body and the sense of self

It is well established that in the not too distant past, women were thought to be controlled (almost entirely) by the uterus; and the relationship of the uterus to the female brain was a common pillar of such thinking. Consequently, many women accepted that their reproductive organs held complete sway over them and they were warned not to divert needed energy away from the uterus and ovaries if they wanted to maintain good health and in fact save their lives. It is said that the upper-class women actively embraced this warning and rested a lot as well as avoided 'brain' work. Women were seen to adopt the stereotype of the invalid and to assume an inferior role simply because that was the 'natural' order — they were sicklier than men because of their biological difference to men (Behar 1991:272–273).

Shorter's (1984) historical account of women's bodies reflects the perceived acceptance of male myths. He claims that there was no protest by women at the subordination of their bodies' biological function and the concomitant subordination of them as menstruating women, pregnant women. However, the means by which women might have exercised resistance to, or evolved an

163

effective voice against such beliefs, makes Shorter's claims somewhat troublesome. This type of history about women's bodies, retrospectively regarded as myth promulgated by men, is likely to have affected women's identity then as it does now, depending on how strongly such views were embodied.

Menstruation marks the commencement of reproductive life, in which case it is a very different stage in a woman's life when it is compared with menopause; yet these two significant biological events have a powerful influence on women's social being and their sense of embodied being. Around the time of menopause women are reminded of their advancing age, whereas the commencement of menstruation signifies growing up — an event about which girls may boast (Gorman & Whitehead 1989 cited by Coney 1991:68–69).

The changes in the biological body at the time referred to as 'mid-life' are very conspicuous both to oneself and others. Whilst women may have had years of social conditioning towards accepting their place in the world, accepting changes in their physical appearance can result in a sadness or type of grieving process. The arrival of lines, 'crow's feet' eyes, grey hair and a changed body shape and size can challenge a woman's view of herself. Why is it significant? The answer in part is the change in social attitude towards women in middle years. There is also a change in attitude towards men but not to the same degree. Men somehow become more distinguished with grey hair and they are often depicted as wiser for their past experience. They are valued for their positions in the workforce and their contributions to society.

There are very definite social images to which a woman of middle years is expected to conform, particularly in her sexual behaviour and her clothing (cf Coney 1991:41–42). A young woman is encouraged to wear 'sexy' body-hugging and revealing clothing that will appeal to the opposite sex. If, however, an older woman wears similar clothing she is accused of not acting her age or may be referred to as 'mutton dressed up as lamb'. The middle-aged woman is supposed to become more invisible and certainly not attract attention in spite of the fact that so many of these women are more confident and self-assured than during their younger years.

Wolf (1990:14) argues that it is precisely the emergence of power in older women that makes them 'unbeautiful'. This may be one factor that affects the social constructions of middle-aged and menopausal women — that power and the female are regarded as mutually exclusive. One of the most difficult things for some women to reconcile in middle age is the view that they are obsolete after menopause, which happens also to coincide with middle age for the majority of women.

The body, social life and meaning-making

Meaning is created by human beings as they interact with one another and with the social and environmental contexts in which they live and how they interpret their experiences. Human experience, while it is strongly influenced by the world, is not dictated or determined by that world. Meaning is contextually constructed by individuals bound both socially and historically.

Shilling (1993:70) says that there is a commonly held premise that the body is 'a receptor, rather than a generator, of social meanings'. This suggests that society somehow has a stronghold over the body — inventing, shaping and constraining it.

There is a strong rejection of the notion that the body can be adequately accounted for as a purely biological phenomenon. It is argued the body is in fact a product of society as individuals embrace particular ideals and meanings of the culture in which they exist and live. Foucault (cited in Shilling 1993:79) for example, argued that 'bodies are highly malleable phenomena which can be invested with various and changing forms of power'. It is these powers that control individuals.

More recently, Turner (1992) has tendered a combined view of the body as a biological organism and as 'lived experience', which contributes towards social relations, albeit with an analysis on the body as a system of representation. The human body, unlike that of animals' bodies, is not programmed to exist and survive within their particular environment. The human world represents little stability, it is not programmed, or pre-set, but relatively open; and it is the individual who must decipher the content and meaning from the human action within their world in order to survive in it.

Shilling (1993:102) says that acceptance of a close alignment between humans and their environment implies 'that human embodiment is an unfinished state which compels people to act on themselves, others and the world around them'. The individual's sense of self and the relation they have with their body is governed by the individual way they process the superabundance of data that presents itself to them. They have to create a meaningful world for themselves.

In recent work on biology and social science, Benton (1991, 1992, reported by Shilling 1993:104–105) argues that we must investigate carefully the inter-relationship between biological and social processes because we will gain some understanding of 'the historical factors' that contribute 'to our current state of embodiment'. He therefore provides support for the view that the body is neither a pre-social, biological phenomenon nor is it a post-biological social entity.

Madjar (1991:52–53), whose work draws on concepts of embodiment derived from Merleau-Ponty, purports that while many valid advances in areas such as biomedicine have occurred, conceiving the body as 'just physical' containing 'measurable properties of mass, weight, size and motion in relation to their objects, is to provide only a partial account of its characteristics and activity'. Gadow (1980:172) describes this conception of the body leading to a final 'disengagement' to a point where the person's body becomes 'a complete abstraction'. Her thesis is that body and self are inseparable but not identical and that the essence of human existence is embodiment.

Merleau-Ponty's work (1962) has contributed much to the development of the sociology of the body and to more generalised works about embodiment. The paradigm view that Merleau-Ponty constructed is summed up in the term 'lived-body', although this term was seldom employed in his original writings. Merleau-Ponty's account of the body is that it is not an object for itself but is 'a spontaneous synthesis of powers, a bodily spatiality, a bodily unity, a bodily intentionality, which distinguish it radically from the scientific object posed by traditional schools of thought' (Langer 1989:56).

Human beings are connected to the world in a unique way, the way we walk, talk and eat are characteristics of our lived body, as perceived to belong to us and no one else. In Merleau-Ponty's words, 'To be a body, is to be tied to a certain world... [because] our body is not primarily *in* space: it is of it' (1962:148). Therefore, if we reduce the human body to mere object states it necessarily becomes inaccessible to lived experience.

Madjar (1991:58–61) uses the work of Benner and Wrubel (1989) to discuss Merleau-Ponty's account of embodiment within five identified dimensions. The first of these is described as an inborn complex that is both pre-personal and pre-cultural, for example thumb sucking in utero. Second is the habitual, skilled body, which refers to those attributes that are socially and culturally acquired, for example eye contact during conversation and the meaning it holds in different cultures. Additionally learnt skills such as driving a car and riding a bicycle are embodied skills, which means we can usually perform them without conscious effort. This dimension becomes problematic when something disrupts the habitual ability of the body that Merleau-Ponty calls the 'body at this moment'. This dimension has particular relevance for individuals in times of illness or, for example, at particular developmental stages of life such as puberty, pregnancy and menopause. The body can feel strange and unfamiliar even distant. There is, however, no male equivalent of these fundamental aspects of women's lives.

The third dimension is the projective body. This refers to the way the body is 'programmed' to move and act. For example, when we walk up or down stairs we do not have to think about how to negotiate each step nor do we concentrate on the depth of each step. The actual projected body is the fourth dimension which is a complex of current projected bodily skills related to a particular skill.

The phenomenal body completes the picture of embodiment and refers to the bodily sensations and body image, that is, the body being aware of itself. The phenomenal body can be experienced with respect to bodily sensations, for example a menopausal hot flush. Women might describe this in a variety of personal and subjective (experienced) ways; the same event can be described, within the objective, biomedical model, as a vasomotor symptom with a physiological basis.

The malleable body: remaking self and body

It is evident that in western society we are witnessing a resurgence of the classical Greek attitudes in relation to the body. The appearance of gyms and fitness centres in large numbers is testimony to what Harré (1986:190) terms the 'fitness freakiness' that has a 'strangle-hold' on both men and women. The fit, athletic body is *that* body to which many aspire and for which they work, exercise and sweat. Cultivation of a society of fitness enthusiasts, in part, is achieved by the ideal body-image portrayed in magazines, on television and all manner of advertising. And we are encouraged by modern health messages to get fit, stay healthy and avoid various lifestyle related conditions.

The implied message is that everyone can achieve the(ir) 'ideal body'. We are being bombarded with messages that promote an image which for most people is more likely the 'unreal body'. There is an inference that to exercise is to display a certain 'moral worth' whereas not engaging in exercise demonstrates a lack of self-control (Harré 1986:191). Striving for the 'ideal body' in whatever form it takes, does not adequately allow for those features of one's physical make-up that are not socially constructed or malleable; for example, in adulthood, one's height is a given, one's skin colour is a given, and one's capacity to redistribute or re-arrange various components that make up body mass are constrained by one's genetic make-up. Where women are concerned, there is not much that one can do to delay or slow the processes of menopause — at least not in relation to existing knowledge about such matters. Yet, the overwhelming message that women receive is to stay young, attractive, slim and sexually desirable.

The body also has become an industry 'with mass consumerism ascribing the signs of appropriate identity' (Carkeek & James 1992). The general expectation that the body should be worked on and reformed through diets, aerobics, plastic surgery and the mode of dress is problematic. In addition, biomedical technologies ascribe various frames for viewing corporeal defects; many body parts are, in the main, replaceable and many 'defects' in the exterior body can be altered by cosmetic surgery.

Bordo (1991) is one of a growing number of authors who are challenging the view that people can or should sculpt their bodies in order to create masterpieces. Yet the power of western science and technology has generated an ideology of the self which is perpetuated through mass culture, which is global and heavily supported by commercial and vested interests. The ideology is also a fuelled by a fantasy that there is no end to the degree of change and improvement thought to be possible in one's body and self.

Embodied self, identity and dysfunctional bodies

Gadow (1980:172) describes the relationship between body and self as inseparable, but not identical, and that embodiment is 'the essence of human existence'. This becomes problematic when we begin to examine embodied self and health related issues when there is a discrepancy between the body as I the patient (the 'I am my body') experience it and the body ('my body') that is treated by medical practitioners and nurses. Gadow proposes that there is a dialectical progression between the self and the body consisting of four levels:

1 primary immediacy: the lived body;
2 disrupted immediacy: the object body;
3 cultivated immediacy: the harmony of the lived body and the object body; and
4 aesthetic immediacy: the subject body, exemplified in ageing and illness.

Primary immediacy (the lived-body experience) has been written about by several philosophers such as Merleau-Ponty, Sartre, Marcel and Ricoeur. The lived body is a positive condition in which I experience my actions as one with myself. It *is* my acting not an instrument with which I act. There is a conscious vulnerability of the lived body, the capacity to experience hurt and injury by the world, and there is no distinction or distance in the relationship between the self and the lived body in primary immediacy. The distinction is that of being aware of the lived body being-in-the-world and the way one is able to affect their world as well as be affected by it.

The self-body unity distinguishes itself from the world and this is its principal focus. This unity is, however, subject to disruption, the break leading to self-distinction. If the self-body is acted upon by a part of itself and not the world, the immediacy of the lived body separates into self and body. The object body emerges as a result of disrupted immediacy.

Disrupted immediacy (the object body) is the second level of self and body relationship in which the self and body are related in the same way as the lived body and world were in primary immediacy. The difference now is that the distinction between agency and vulnerability is internal as opposed to external. It is the body and self acting upon each other in place of the lived body and world interaction in the first level. The lived body immediacy is shattered and the self is now opposed to the body. The body can become constrained by illness, disability or biological experiences such as puberty, menopause and ageing. The resultant relationship is one of a struggle between the body and self as they conflict with one another.

Strauss (1987:203) refers to the continuity of self and body as a biographical body conception chain, which can be broken by illness that results in a failed body. The process is an unconscious one involving the senses of sight, smell, sound, touch and taste and the perceptions we form through these. When the chain is interrupted by a failed body we can no longer play out our biography.

There are many examples of chronic illnesses and injury where the links of the chain are broken, for example chronic renal failure, stroke and heart disease. When a person experiences chronic renal failure the relationship between their body and self can be interrupted by a change in the way they see themselves. The colour and condition of their skin may change and they may have to reintegrate and reconstruct the self to embody a change in self and identity. The person may face the situation of dialysis as it becomes an essential part of their life when their biological body fails them. The embodied taken-for-grantedness of the body's biological function is replaced with an awareness of its susceptibility to breakdown.

The image of a failing body requires a change within the person. They will need to incorporate a new body image into a revised self-identity — that is, they will develop a new sense of embodiment. Martin (1987:19) proposes that this is even more evident if the person were to have a renal transplant. This, as with any transplantation of body parts, will lead to numerous readjustments in self-concept and in one's sense of relationship to fellow humans.

The new relation between body and self in the example is the inversion of the self as master, a free subjectivity rendering the self a slave to the rebelling body. Inevitably, in this type of situation, body and self are at odds with one another. There is an ambiguous freedom and bondage between self and body with one either being controlled or controlling the other. This body is now out of synchrony or harmony and is the existential otherness of the self — the object body. To use Gadow's words, 'the object body emerges out of the primary unity of the lived body in the experience of feeling encumbered by oneself' (1980:176).

When concepts of self and identity are ruptured in cases of illness, disease and injury, the person will attempt to restore unity of the self and the body, which can take two directions. The first leads to a new dichotomy and the second a new unity. The first direction reproduces or re-enacts the master servant dialectic with the production of the theoretical object body of the sciences. In this instance, the self attempts to master the body by objectifying it and comprehending it scientifically. We actively engage in this dichotomous behaviour when we visit a medical practitioner and talk about our body in an objective disembodying manner. Heidegger (1962:95–107) says that as long as our bodily function is in good order, that is 'ready-to-hand', it is overlooked. The sick body is no longer one ready-to-hand and can be experienced in varying degrees of useability. Something is missing and it may refuse to do what it once was capable of and is now just 'present-at-hand'.

The second direction involves an attempt to recover the concrete unity of self and body. The body is not mastered but there is an articulation between self and body with recovery of the original unity albeit at a new level. Gadow (1980:177–178) uses the term 'cultivated immediacy' to describe the restoration of harmony of the lived body and the object body. We might use the example here of a person who has had a stroke and is unable to walk without the aid of a walking stick. This person may struggle initially with the act of walking — the body refusing to perform at will or on command even though prior to the stroke this person would probably never have consciously thought about the act of walking per se. The lived body is taken for granted in that we can move around at will or, as with this example, walk without thinking about how it is that we can lift our feet, what muscles are involved, the nerve pathways involved and the support the skeleton provides in the act of walking. Oliver Sacks (1984) has articulated this phenomenon explicitly in his personal account of the extreme difficulty he faced in taking the first step following a severe leg injury.

Walking, like may embodied acts, is an habitual experience until something disrupts the unity between self and body (e.g. Sacks' experience). A deliberate effort at mastering a new naturalness has to be effected if the limitation brought about by the loss of habitual bodily acts is to be transcended. In other words, the self must re-establish mastery over the body to overcome biologically produced limitations. Leder (1990:80–81) argues that following a stroke or heart attack the person will not want to look to the future because the landscape is seen not as a field of opportunities and possibility but as a field of difficulties to negotiate.

The process of bodily objectification is examined by Leder (1984:34–35) in relation to the encounter with the medical practitioner. He argues that from the doctor's first patient encounter, often a cadaver, she/he primarily comes to see the physical body and lived embodiment is disregarded or at best given token attention. The focus is on diagnosis of disease, the physical locus of pathology, and they are driven by their need or desire to 'cure'.

The sense of the body as an alien thing does not arise solely with the person presenting her/himself to the practitioner. The person may have come to regard their own body as object as a result of the illness process, injury, or pain having caused a split between the body and the self as one's own corporeality exhibits a foreign will. The painful or disabled body no longer appears to be one with the self but is exterior or Other. Similarly, we never escape the lived body even though we can become alienated from our physical body. It may be that at certain periods of serious illness we intentionally alienate the essential self from the body to enable the self to cope with invasive procedures.

In times of serious illness, the body may be temporarily placed fully in the care of the medical practitioner and nurse. Leder (1990:69–99) uses the concept of the 'dys-appearing body' to discuss the body's emergence from disappearance to thematic object in cases of pain and disease, this is, bringing corporeality to explicit awareness for the sufferer.

A study by Price (1993:49–50) in relation to one's physical self-awareness in chronic illness reveals some significant factors that highlight the link between the individual's perception of self and their body. A history of past illness experiences may be relatively insignificant but what has been embodied as a result of an illness may have long-term consequences. For example, people with asthma may consider themselves to be 'allergic types' who are vulnerable to illness; or a person may self identify as a member of a family prone to headaches and individually embody this biographical body conception.

Western approaches to health care have promoted a disease orientation model in which the physical body is the site of pathology. Hadd (1991:168) asserts that using the analogy of body as a machine and separate from the mind is to 'deny our humanity' and 'our personality'. As a model, western medicine has not accommodated the lived body, and it has marginalised embodied experiences as central features of the experience of illness or bodily malfunctions. This is particularly apparent in the case of the medicalisation of menopause.

Menopause as an embodied experience

Women's experience of menopause, as an illustrative example, clearly shows that the body is both a biological and experienced entity, imbued with social values that have been embodied by individuals and sexualised in our culture. The body of a menopausal woman is often regarded as purely a biological body, particularly in relation to the discourses and practices adopted by the medical profession. For women experiencing menopause, the body is much more than a physical entity.

What does it mean to be menopausal? The answer to this question will depend on who is asked and when it is asked; the answers will be different for men and women as well as for individuals. There are medical views in which menopause is defined as a deficiency disease state such that everything a woman experiences is attributed to biology. Other views, such as those of feminists (see for example, Callaway 1981, MacPherson 1981, McCrea 1983, Dickson 1990 and Greer 1991), claim that menopause is a natural event in life like other developmental processes.

Grosz (1990) however, highlights the difficulty we face when we try to decipher meanings embodied in biology. It is not sufficient to simply provide a biological explanation of menopause; nor is it sufficient to rely only on social explanations and 'normalising' discourses for an adequate account of the experience of menopause in western culture. By the time women reach the average age at which menopause occurs — said to be 51 years in Australia (Eden 1992:14) — they have had a lifetime of exposure to social messages that shape beliefs and expectations about menopause and its multiple meanings.

The female, glamour, age, sex, and desirability

Glamour and beauty have long been associated with the young and in western society one generally does not look forward to being an older person, particularly if one is a woman — an attitude that Wolf (1990:10) calls a 'terror of aging'. The very dim view of the older woman — coupled with the very negative attitudes and beliefs about menopause as an experience and the menopausal woman — can affect the way women's concept of self and identity are formed.

The youthful body is seen as a productive body. Historically, and in different ways, patriarchal western society creates a problem for women because their roles have been constructed by and reinforced or mediated through their body and its ability to reproduce. Martin (1987:46–49), for example, has shown how 'an information-transmitting system with a hierarchical structure' typically is used to portray menstruation and menopause in medical texts. What Martin found in examining medical texts is also clearly apparent in nursing texts. The biological control the reproductive system has over the body is likened to the dominant form of organisation in our society, including numerous metaphors of the distribution of power and of production. The language used in describing the physiological processes of women's reproductive functioning is about control over the body. That control is located in a signal system in which the hypothalamus is credited as the master, receiving information from the body and in turn controlling the menstrual cycle. Although there is a feedback system from the hypothalamus to the pituitary to the ovary and back again, the hypothalamus is usually described as being in charge.

Estok and O'Toole (1991:36) cite some of McCrea's (1983) earlier work in which she examined the medical definition of menopause and isolated four themes arising from it. They are:

1 that potential and function are biologically destined;
2 that worth is determined by reproductive ability and attractiveness;
3 that physical and emotional havoc will result from a rejection of the feminine role;
4 that ageing women are repulsive and useless.

It is not difficult to see that if women accept these ideas and images the subject of menopause may not be discussed openly because people find it embarrassing — as Masling (1988:35) has suggested. And if we hold the view of the female body as one that is primarily designed for production and that the female's existence is primarily for reproduction, we will foster the portrayal of women as victims of their reproductive anatomy, which Shorter (1984) has explored in depth.

If sexuality, femininity and being a woman are expressed as being fundamentally tied to the reproductive organs and reproductive experience, then the way in which women and men view menopause (and infertility) is problematic from the perspective of women's experiences of self and body. In cases of infertility and unexpected menopause the woman may feel let down or failed by her body. When the familiar and often highly predictable changes that signal to individuals that their body is in its regular cycling pattern become disrupted, the sense of the customary body and the body at the moment is also disrupted.

Reaction to this disruption to the body's normal pattern may be fear of losing control as the embodied self undergoes novel sensations and altered capacities. If menstruation signals the capacity to reproduce, the cessation of menstruation renders the body unproductive; and the discourses and language used to describe the female reproductive system once it becomes unproductive are imbued with negativity. The vagina 'atrophies', 'declines', 'shrinks' and the ovaries are said to be 'senile' or 'insufficient'. There are no equivalent words or terms used to describe changes in the male reproductive system; but there is also no male equivalent of the menopause.

It is argued by some that the medicalisation of menopause is an attempt to uphold male power and control over women (MacPherson 1981, Reitz 1985, Martin 1987, Greer 1991). Behar (1991:274) cites the readiness to perform hysterectomies on either malfunctioning or ageing wombs as evidence of the disdain for a non-productive menopausal body. Embodying this vision of menopause not only propagates the current social order but can block any alternative view(s).

Medical practitioners view the uterus as an unimportant organ if the woman no longer wants to have children or she is 'past it' in terms of having reached the socially acceptable age to bear children. It is common practice, among some surgeons, to remove the woman's ovaries at the same time as their uterus if they do not look healthy at the time of surgery or because of the small risk of developing ovarian cancer. Again, there is no male comparison with this type of surgery, nor is there any similar 'logic' that is applied to male reproductive functioning; rather, there is no age limit at which a man is said to 'past it' in a reproductive sense. The sense of embodied womanliness or wholeness, as an individual, is not factored into constructs about the usefulness or value of women's reproductive organs.

It seems ironic that we have moved so little from the grim stereotype of menopausal women originally outlined by Wilson and Wilson (1963) and Wilson (1966). They made explicit the concept of menopause as a disease in which women are destined to a sort of living decay without hormone replacement therapy. The idea that menopause is a sex-linked, hereditary, oestrogen deficiency disease continues to be promoted by various groups.

What belief women hold about menopause, as well as the views of those they consult, will affect the way they respond to it and the way they respond to others who are menopausal; and it will affect the ways they relate to their own bodies and their sense of being an embodied woman. Women who may be exposed only to the disease model of menopause may expect to have an awful time and those who come to regard it as a normal event in life, just like other stages, may not dread its coming but, as Greer contends, actually welcome it.

Greer (1991:46) presents an alternative view to the one which argues that in middle age a woman is afraid of not continuing to function as a responsive lover, dutiful wife and valuable efficient employee. On the contrary, she says that these women may not want to continue fulfilling these roles and dares to suggest they may be actually tired of it all. If we are within an environment that silences matters such as menopause, then we are more likely not to discuss any symptoms.

In the 1990s we have witnessed a change in the taboos associated with discussing topics such as menopause. What was once a forbidden and silent topic is now being discussed more openly by politicians, mayors and women who have high social profiles (e.g. Liechti 1993 has contributions from many prominent Australian women). Holding these women up as examples of successful women who also happen to be menopausal, may help to dispel the myth that older or ageing women are useless or that their worth is determined by fecundity. It may also perpetuate the view that these women are powerful and in control and that they therefore do not (and apparently can not) represent the 'average' woman.

Summary

Humans are, by definition, embodied and they are individually embodied. But as social beings, their sense of embodiment is heavily imbued with social, historical and cultural meanings. In the context of health care, disruptions to normal body patterning, dysfunctions of their bodies and individual experiences are shaped by and partly dependent on wider concepts of the ideal(ised) self, embodied individuality and physical form. The concept of self, which is affected by the biological body, however, is not necessarily dependent on physicality.

While humans are, to a large extent, biologically determined and constrained by their bodies, so too are they constrained by, or able to transcend, personal and socially constructed meanings about what their bodies represent

REFERENCES

Behar R 1991 The body in the woman: a book review and personal essay. In: Goldstein L (ed) The female body. University of Michigan Press, Michigan
Bordo S 1990 Reading the slender body. In: Jacobs M (ed) Body/politics: women and the discourses of science. Routledge & Kegan Paul, London, 83–112

Bordo S 1991 'Material girl': the effacements of postmodern culture. In: Goldstein L (ed) The female body. University of Michigan Press, Michigan, 106–130

Callaway H 1981 Women's perspectives: research as re-vision. In: Reason P, Rowan J (eds) Human inquiry. Wiley, New York

Carkeek F, James P 1992 The self, the body and identity. Arena (99/100):66–85

Coney S 1991 The menopause industry. Spinifex, Melbourne

Descartes R 1986 Discourse on method and the meditations. Penguin, Harmondsworth

Dickson G 1990 A feminist poststructuralist analysis of the knowledge of menopause. Advances in Nursing Science 12(3):15– 31

Eden J 1992 Women's hormone problems. The Royal Hospital for Women, Paddington

Elias N 1985 The civilizing process: the history of manners. Blackwell, Oxford

Estok P, O'Toole R 1991 The meanings of menopause. Health Care for Women International 12:27–39

Gadow S 1980 Body and self: a dialectic. The Journal of Medicine and Philosophy 5(3):172–185

Game A 1991 Undoing the social: towards a deconstructive sociology. Open University Press, Milton Keynes

Greer G 1991 The change. Hamish Hamilton, London

Grosz E 1990 A note on essentialism and difference. In: Gunew S (ed) Feminist knowledge: critique and construct. Routledge, London, 332–344

Grosz E 1994 Volatile bodies. Allen & Unwin, Sydney

Hadd W 1991 A womb with a view: women as mothers and the discourse of the body. Berkeley Journal of Sociology 36:165–175

Harré R 1986 Is the body a thing? International Journal of Moral and Social Studies 1(3):188–203

Heidegger M 1962 Being and time. Translated by J Macquarrie and E Robinson. Blackwell, Oxford

Langer M 1989 Merleau-Ponty's phenomenology of perception: a guide and commentary. Macmillan Press, London

Lawler J 1991 Behind the screens: nursing, somology, and the problem of the body. Churchill Livingstone, Melbourne

Leder D 1984 Medicine and paradigms of embodiment. The Journal of Medicine and Philosophy 9(1):29–44

Leder D 1990 The absent body. The University of Chicago Press, Chicago

Leonard V W 1989 A Heideggerian phenomenologic perspective on the concept of the person. Advances in Nursing Science 11(4):40–55

Liechti Y 1993 A new start. Sally Milner, Sydney

MacPherson K I 1981 Menopause as disease: the social construction of a metaphor. Advances in Nursing Science 3(2)95–113

Madjar I 1991 Pain as an embodied experience: a phenomenological study of clinically inflicted pain in adult patients. PhD thesis, Massey University

Martin E 1987 The woman in the body. Beacon Press, Boston

Masling J 1988 Menopause a change for the better? Nursing Times 84 (39): 35-38

McCrea F 1983 The politics of menopause: 'discovery' of a deficiency disease. Social Problems 31 (1): 111-123

Merleau-Ponty M 1962 The phenomenology of perception. Translated by Colin Smith. Routledge & Kegan Paul, London

Morgan D H J, Scott S 1993 Bodies in a social landscape. In: Scott S, Morgan D H J (eds) Body matters. Falmer Press, London, 1–21

Price M J 1993 Exploration of body listening: health and physical self-awareness in chronic illness. Advances in Nursing Science 15(4):37–52

Reiger K 1987 The embodiment of resistance: reproductive struggles and feminism. Arena (79):92–107

Reitz R 1985 Menopause a positive approach. Unwin, London

Sacks O 1984 A leg to stand on. Harper and Row, New York

Sheets-Johnstone M 1992 Charting the interdisciplinary course. In: Sheets-Johnstone M (ed) Giving the body its due. New York Press, Albany, 1–15

Shilling C 1993 The body and social theory. Sage, London

Shorter E 1984 A history of women's bodies. Penguin, Middlesex

Strauss A L 1987 Qualitative analysis for social scientists. Cambridge University Press, Cambridge

Synnott A 1993 The body social. Routledge, London

The Australian Oxford pocket dictionary 1986 Turner G (ed). Oxford University Press, Melbourne

Turner B S 1992 Regulating bodies. Routledge, London

Wilson R, Wilson T 1963 The fate of the nontreated postmenopausal woman: a plea for the maintenance of adequate oestrogen from puberty to the grave. Journal of the American Geriatric Society 11:347–362

Wilson R 1966 Feminine forever. Allen, London

Wolf N 1994 The beauty myth. Vintage, London

Zaner R M 1964 The problem of embodiment. Martinus Nijhoff, The Hague

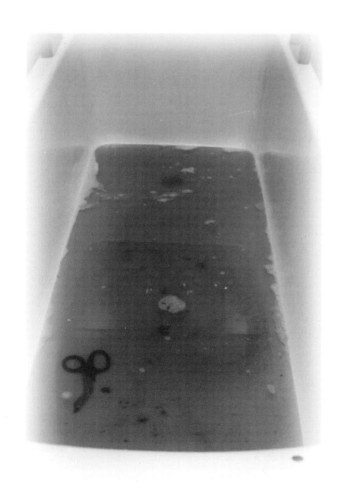

11

Some consequences of the psychiatric dis-integration of the body, mind and soul

Jan Horsfall

Introduction

In this chapter I investigate psychiatric nursing epistemologies and their medical origins. After clarifying the specific material underpinnings of the discipline, I discuss factors which are excluded from such ways of knowing. Human qualities, which could be described as soul, along with emotions and lived experience, are missing from both material (physical bodily) and rational (mind-cognitive) models of psychiatry. Furthermore, I argue that these have negative consequences for the agency of the nurse and the client.

I have chosen to explore psychiatric states called 'depressions', because definitions of these include a number of bodily phenomena. Such conditions may allow investigators to discern the assumed or articulated relationships between body and mind within mainstream psychiatry. I will also discuss schizophrenias, because psychiatry does not necessarily claim that these disorders display bodily signs. By investigating both depressions and schizophrenias I hope to include a broad range of psychiatric phenomena (neurotic and psychotic) in this essay.

Psychiatric disorders as symbols of social fears

What does the pathologised spectre called depression hold? According to contemporary psychiatric diagnosis criteria (American Psychiatric Association 1994), depression includes lowered mood, diminished pleasure, insomnia, slow movements, fatigue, guilty beliefs, difficulty in concentration and thoughts of death. I argue that each of these is a socio-culturally determined problem or anxiety (Horsfall 1994a:172–175). From this aggregation of human phenomena, it seems that mainstream western society fears or forbids misery, sloth, tiredness and the reality of our inevitable death.

The physical body invoked in this medical description of depression symptoms is implicitly a faulty body if not an incapacitated body. In depression it seems that this faulty body is not sleeping properly, it is travelling at an inappropriately slow pace, it is tired, it feels burdened and heavy. Depression presses upon the body. The depressed body is neither consuming nor producing in ways it should be in a capitalist society. At the more superficial level, this body is disruptive in that it is not seducing, nor is it seducible: it ignores pleasures, sensuality, sex and it is blatantly failing to have fun. It is not a healthy, aesthetically fit body, it displays lethargy and sloth. The depressed body cannot be the ideal maternal body because it has insufficient energies to enfold, forgive, nurture or invest in others. The depressed body cannot house the ideal reliable and busy multiskilled worker. Furthermore, a depressed person's face is not the stereotypical social face we expect, instead it is expressionless, immobile and fails to be polite.

In depression, the mind is also faulty. It is not concentrating and it is thinking too much about the wrong things: a certain amount of privately undermining guilt is acceptable as are silent fears about mortality. However, to proclaim at length and loudly to the world that one is guilty of omissions and commissions is often annoying to others; and to ruminate about the advantages of, and articulate a preference for, death is unnerving and disturbing to those who inhabit the space around the depressed person. The depressed mind is not lively, interesting or distracting, the voice that emerges from this state is flat and the words are often monosyllabic and gloomy.

Symbolically, depression can be seen to be an affront to our ideals of sociability, gendered behaviours and commitments to work and money. By discussing depression in these ways I do not dispute or deny the pain, entrapment and suffering which depressed people experience (cf. Ussher 1991:220–221). However it is clear from my social and interpersonal reading of depression (over two decades of clinical experience), that it must be extremely difficult for depressed persons to gain the sort of respect, support, and understanding they usually need from nurses or any other health workers.

Depressions reveal certain socially stigmatised attitudes of body and mind. The schizophrenias do not necessarily display bodily disturbances: the mind offers more of a focus for medical interests in this instance. Of all of the psychiatric syndromes discussed by lay people, schizophrenia is the condition most imbued with fear. What qualities has the discipline of psychiatry gathered together under this label, which renders this the most terrifying of psychiatric problems? People who live through a psychotic episode commonly experience terror, identity disintegration, fear of madness, anguish, extreme distrust of others and perceptual confusion. In other words, lay connotations of fear and terror match, albeit to a lesser extent, the lived experiences of the hallucinating person.

A more technical description of schizophrenic symptoms (American Psychiatric Association 1994) includes delusions — the adherence to specific beliefs that can usually be shown to be not supportable according to evidence from a range of other people or sources. The other primary symptom is that of hallucinations, which are idiosyncratic sensory distortions that most other people have not experienced and have difficulty even imagining. These beliefs and perceptions may become sufficiently intrusive so that the person cannot participate meaningfully in a conversation, misreads ordinary social conventions and is not in a fit state to carry out work for hours on end in predictable ways (cf. Maguire 1992:217). Once these experiences reach a critical pitch, daily living is severely impeded.

Unlike depression, where many of the 'symptoms' can be seen as bodily manifestations, this reading is not apparent for most schizophrenias. Most of the human phenomena clustered together and named schizophrenia relate rather more to the mind. Thinking, perceiving, judging and believing are interfered with. Speaking, conversing and interacting are disrupted in response to the interior hallucinations or delusions. Common further responses to the internal bombardment and confusion are social isolation, inattention to basic activities such as personal hygiene and adequate nutrition; as well as a comprehensive disruption of the diurnal rhythm of daily living.

Here the body seems to be implicated with regard to the possibilities of acting out unusual behaviours, which are related to disturbing thoughts or perceptual experiences — the transparent body revealing its inner secrets (cf. Grosz 1994:9). However, like the depressed body, the schizophrenic body may be marked by anergia, impaired mobility and an implacable asocial face. The schizophrenic body is far removed from any of the socially idealised bodies; it is not lively, energetic or fit; it is not fun loving; and it cannot predicably focus on, or carry through with, work or parenting activities.

In this section of the chapter I have briefly outlined my hermeneutic understandings of the psychiatric conditions known as depression and schizophrenia. I have tried to read these designated disorders from a perspective that allows for social meanings rather than medical description or reductivist symptoms. My aim is to destabilise and deconstruct these psychiatric disorders (as specific exemplars) to the extent that their inevitability and existence as medical problems is questioned. The vulnerabilities (cf. Vines 1993) revealed by such an examination indicate anxieties regarding work and social interactions, and at another level, anxieties about death, personal identity and alternative 'realities'.

Medico-psychiatric hegemony

The medical-psychiatric way of looking at these human experiences is hegemonic amongst the great majority of nurses and other health workers (cf. Pilgrim & Treacher 1992:1), clients of the psychiatric sector, friends and family members as well as the public in general. This epistemological stranglehold has prevailed for over a century in European countries and is increasingly invading other societies whose peoples have held different beliefs about these human maladies.

Given these circumstances, it is imperative to propose interpretations, descriptions, models or theories to counter the present psychiatric system of naming, medicating and disposing of patients. The medical belief system has been briefly challenged this century by psychoanalysis, Laing's (1960) existential psychiatry, certain schools of family therapy, and by feminists. De-radicalised psychoanalysis and gestures towards family therapy insights have been colonised by psychiatry and incorporated into the discipline. Laing's works were attacked, discredited and discarded, those of feminism have mostly been ignored, but are sometimes misinterpreted and discounted. This leaves mainstream psychiatry in charge of the practices and ideologies associated with named and described psychiatric conditions.

In the next section I examine a psychiatric nursing text to ascertain the extent to which medical knowledge dominates nursing understandings of bodies and minds of people who experience depressions and schizophrenias.

Mainstream nursing understandings of schizophrenias and depressions

I am using Wilson and Kneisl's (1992) well-known US psychiatric nursing text, *Psychiatric Nursing*, as an exemplar, because it starkly reveals the underlying assumptions about the human body and mind which prevail in mental health nursing in English speaking countries in the 1990s. It is also a relatively typical example of psychiatric nursing texts.

In the first chapter of the text the reader is informed that in this 'decade of the brain' scientific and technological research into 'brain dysfunction' in schizophrenias has leapt ahead.

> As researchers have discovered a variety of brain dysfunctions, including ventricular enlargement, cerebral atrophy, and disturbances in neurotransmitters, treatment approaches for schizophrenia became more differentiated. The outcome is less emphasis on providing psychotherapy and more emphasis on achieving social rehabilitation (Wilson & Kneisl 1992:15).

Scientists are using imaging technologies to shore up claims that the faulty body is the primary cause of schizophrenias. However once the body has been blamed, the social consequences must be rectified!

Even though a medley of models (including analytic, psychological and nursing frameworks) has been introduced, it is clear that the medical 'psychobiologic' model has practical and ideological priority. However, some nursing authors (Abraham, Fox & Cohen 1992:296) go so far as to state that biology is radically under-valued in mental health nursing. Wilson and Kneisl (1992) promote the psychobiological model enthusiastically, but to some extent this is obfuscated. They claim (for example) that 'psychiatric diagnoses according to DSM-III-R [the international medical-psychiatric diagnostic manual] are based on specified, empirical criteria not linked to any particular theory or etiology' (Wilson & Kneisl 1992:62). Such statements may indicate that mental health nurses do not overtly adhere to the ideologies of the medico-psychiatric model, but simply follow its pragmatic treatment consequences.

According to McEnany (in Wilson & Kneisl 1992:100) psychobiology is

> the study of the biochemical foundations of thought, mood, emotion, affect, and behaviour. It takes into consideration both internal and external

influences — e.g. genetics, the effects of other body systems such as the endocrine and immune systems, and the external environment.

This is not only a claim to scientific explanations of psychiatric conditions, but a claim to an understanding of the complexities of human thinking, feeling(s) and behaviour(s). This is about the cerebrum, thalamus, hypothalamus, cerebellum, brain stem, neurones and neurotransmitters. The material is an abridged neuroanatomy, electrochemistry and psychoendocrinology which is then applied to all major psychiatric conditions.

After declaring that the dopamine hypothesis is 'the most probable explanation' of schizophrenias, McEnany (1992:114) states that 'changes in cortisol regulation yield the **vegetative signs of depression** and include symptoms such as psychomotor retardation, anorexia, constipation, lethargy, diminished libido, poor concentration, and insomnia' (cf. Wilson & Kneisl 1992:260, emphasis in original). This is presented not as an hypothesis, but as an hormonal basis for specific medical symptoms of depression. To put these types of claims into perspective, one is forced to leave psychiatric nursing literature.

Vines (1993:55) notes that 'different studies have reported low melatonin levels and high cortisol levels in depressed or schizophrenic patients, but the evidence continues to be poor'. She also points to a more invidious aspect of such scientific wishful thinking, that is, the greater the focus on psycho-endocrinology, the less focus there is on sufferers' social worlds (Vines 1993:55).

Even within psychoendocrinology, the roles of specific hormones are unclear. McEnany lists 'conditions that result from disordered peptide [a hormonal class] functioning'. From this, depression may be related to hypercortisolism, hypocortisolism, hypothyroidism and autoimmune thyroiditis; and prolactin is implicated in relation to lethargy (1992:109).

What are Wilson and Kneisl saying about schizophrenias and depressions? I note that they say very little about the lived experiences of the persons, their bodies, their minds, their feelings, their voiced concerns or desires.

Medical researchers seem to be determined that neurotransmitters are at the bottom of our most socially feared psychiatric disorders. As the purported connections between depressions and cortisol (or other hormones) is a long-shot, so too is the proclaimed close connection between dopamine (or other neurotransmitters) and schizophrenias. McEnany (1992:108) states that:

> dopamine is a plentiful neurotransmitter synthesised from dietary amino acid tyrosine and found in three parts of the brain: the brain's substantial nigra motor centre (affecting movement and coordination), the midbrain (involving emotion and memory), and the hypothalamus/pituitary connection (involving emotional responses and stress-coping patterns).

In other words, dopamine is involved in many of our ordinary human capacities. Some people with a schizophrenic diagnosis have no coordination difficulties (beyond medication effects), no memory impediment or no unusual emotional responses, given the gravity of the disorder.

Ultimately Wilson and Kneisl's (1992) psychiatric nursing text primarily provides a neurotransmitter (electrochemical) explanation of schizophrenias (p.260) and depressions (pp.288,291) with an overlay of hormones (pp.291–292) in the latter. The schizophrenias are assumed to be underpinned by 'genetic vulnerabilities' (p.260) which are also implicated in the depressions (p.288). Readers are reminded that these two biological stalwarts — genes and hormones — are often invoked as determinants of human differences, including gender (Birke 1992:66) and sexual orientation (Vines 1993:113–115).

Generally the mental health nursing texts re-present the medico-psychiatric picture of psychiatric conditions. Such a model has narrow and instrumental 'treatment' consequences. But at a more fundamental level these aetiological schemata convey specific ideological messages about people's minds and bodies: in health as well as in disturbance.

In the next sections of the chapter I set out and critique the genetic and electrochemical view of the body and mind in more detail. Both models are reductionist and deterministic. According to dictionary definitions, the mind is the focus of the discipline of psychiatry; and these hegemonic models disintegrate the mind as much as the body.

The genetically determined body and mind

Biological determinism finds its most eloquent expression in the genetic view of health and disease. The medical-scientific drive to locate a genetic cause of schizophrenias and depressions has been evident for about a century and this tradition derives from the dominant (both medically and socially in European countries) nineteenth century belief in heredity and degeneration, especially when applied to the lower classes. A materialist understanding (one which eschews soul, emotions and social factors) of psychiatric disorders has gained momentum within medicine since Cullen's mid-eighteenth century recourse to Cartesian philosophy and Newtonian science (Horsfall 1994a:47); and it has peaked in the last quarter of this century.

The original work on the proclaimed genetic causation of schizophrenias, which continues to be cited, is that of Kallman whose data were collected between 1893 and 1902 — before schizophrenia was actually named (Horsfall 1994a:101–102)! One likely consequence of the name change from dementia praecox to schizophrenia in 1911 is the lack of clear and unequivocal definition of schizophrenia. According to Gilman (1988:227), Kallman claimed that schizophrenics were 'an increasing source of maladjusted cranks, social eccentrics and the lowest type of criminal offenders'. When he left Germany and set up the first genetics research institute in the USA his interest in eugenics did not necessarily diminish.

The research design, which is deemed to provide the best scientific evidence that specific conditions are genetically inherited, is that of twin studies. Concordance rates for schizophrenia (i.e. the presence or absence of schizophrenia) are consistently higher for monozygotic twins (those with the same genetic inheritance) than it is for dizygotic twins (Wilson & Kneisl 1992:260). Apart from any other confounding factors in relation to sampling, analysis or interpretation of monozygotic twin studies, disorder definitions is a significant problem. In a recent study of over one thousand female twin pairs, the team of geneticists and psychiatrists problematised depression symptoms and found that — depending on the definition — the 'estimated heritability of genetic liability' for depression ranged from twenty-one to forty-five per cent (Kendler et al 1992). Needless to say, the tighter the definition the lower the estimated genetic heritability. Kallman's 'maladjusted cranks' provided a suitably vague category which would easily allow him to appear to prove that schizophrenia, so defined (or not defined), is inherited via 'defective' family genes.

In the genetic schema, the body and mind are, by implication, reduced to determinant inherited matter. Within this modus operandi, medical researchers reduce a complex bodily-emotional-social state such as depression to a faulty code in the basic building blocks of living creatures.

Electrochemical orchestration of body and mind

Genetics is not the only example of psychiatric reductionism in relation to the human body and mind. The more modern focus on neurotransmitters is another fine example. Within the European medical materialist tradition, the body has been understood as a series of 'systems', which are commonly studied as entities, somewhat distinct from each other. Conventional medical specialities attest to these, for example cardiovascular, respiratory or endocrinology specialists are deemed to have separate domains of expertise.

The central nervous system is one of these 'systems'. This complex and powerful system is often reduced to the brain, which is then imbued with an actual, and symbolic, significance in its own right. As early as the 1830s, Griesinger made the following claims that are not out of place in 1990s psychiatry.

> We therefore, primarily, and in every case of mental disease, recognize a morbid action of that organ [the brain]... . Pathology proves as clearly as physiology, that the brain alone can be the seat of normal and abnormal mental action' (cited in Jackson 1986:163).

Contrary to nineteenth century expectations that specific cerebral sites would yield answers to psychiatric, as well as neurological symptomatology, this has not been the case.

Consequently, medical researchers have been forced, in accordance with the imperative that the brain must hold these secrets, into even more microscopic reductionism. The central nervous system has become the brain, and the brain — beyond the physical lobes and designated cortical regions — is reduced to nerve cells (neurons), axons and gaps (synapses) between cells. Then the study narrows even further to the neurotransmitters, which chemically facilitate the transmission of electrical charges across the synapses.

At this level, it eventually becomes clear to the researchers that neurotransmitters do not work in isolation from other neurochemicals. In fact hormones may co-exist with, and apparently perform like, neurotransmitters.

183

'The peptides function as neurotransmitters, i.e. they assist in neurotransmission but are not solely responsible for the entire biochemical synaptic sequence' (McEnany 1992:109).

According to the medical neurotransmitter model, the body — in sickness and in health — responds to the commands of neurons and hormones. In this schema the body is material, and matter is manifest as pre-set mechanisms which ultimately determine our emotions, perceptions, motor coordination, madness etc. Consequently the mind and emotions are reduced to the elements of the central nervous system and hormones, that is, to psychoendocrinology.

The dis-integrated mind

In the previous two sections of this chapter I argue that medical, nursing and lay models of the bodies and minds of 'normal' and 'abnormal' people are reduced to genetics and neurotransmitters. The dis-integration of the *soma* (body) into separate systems is paralleled by the modern dis-integration of the psyche. As one does not find the (whole) body in the mental health nursing texts, neither can one find the (whole) mind, let alone a person.

The mind in mainstream medicine and psychology is commonly reduced to specified human attributes, viz. cognitions, perceptions and emotions. Even these fragments are difficult to trace in psychiatric nursing texts. In Wilson and Kneisl's (1992:158–160) text, for example, attenuated aspects of emotions, perceptions, memory and cognition appear dispersed under the umbrella of the mental status examination — a procedure claimed by psychiatrists, psychologists as well as mental health nurses.

A contemporary psychological schema which purports to understand the mind — of well and disturbed people — is the cognitive model. This framework is the perfect complement of the material medical model: each falls on one side of the Cartesian body-mind dualism. The physical schema ultimately considers our bodies to be our destinies and in control of emotions, perceptions and cognitions. The cognitive schema considers our wilful minds to be in control of ideas, beliefs and attitudes (usually considered to be illogical or erroneous), which seriously impact (usually negatively) on our emotions and behaviours. Like the medical model adherents, the proponents of the cognitive model make grand claims for their perspective and the treatments that support them.

> The goals of cognitive therapy are to correct faulty information processing and to help patients modify assumptions that maintain maladaptive behaviours and emotions. Cognitive and behavioural methods are used to challenge dysfunctional beliefs and to promote more realistic adaptive thinking (Beck & Weishaar cited in Ussher 1991:97).

As Ussher (1991:115) points out, cognitive models and treatments have been applied to people who experience depression, anxiety and schizophrenia as well as those who may be distressed or have interpersonal difficulties. However, Aaron Beck — a founding father — began, and continues most of his work, in the area of depression and cognitive therapists mostly do not intend to work with people who have schizophrenic experiences. The basic claim is that the misery, guilt and inertia of depression are caused by self-devaluing beliefs, ruminative negative thoughts and pessimistic self-fulfilling prophecies. As with the medical model, there is no credit given to the person's lived experiences of being actively devalued by family members or society in general, of internalising those beliefs, or of finding that it is impossible to change one's confining external circumstances.

The contemporary cognitive model is as reductive as its physical counterpart. Both elevate an aspect of human reality to the status of an essence — on either side of the Cartesian body-mind divide. Cartesian dualisms have permeated mainstream European sciences and philosophy during the last three centuries. Consequently western medicine is marked by the mind-body divide at both epistemological and practice levels. Naturally psychiatry, as a medical specialty, has inherited this division.

In Grosz's (1994:7) view:

> Rationalism and idealism are the results of the attempt to explain the body and matter in terms of mind, ideas, or reason; empiricism and materialism are the results of attempts to explain the mind in terms of bodily experiences or matter.

Medicine has opted for materialist 'explanations' of psychiatric conditions. Mental health nursing has followed.

Materialist medicine and psychiatric nursing

Psychiatric nursing has largely uncritically taken up this materialist position. McEnany for example, declares that 'the brain provides the underlying biology for will, determination, hopes, and dreams' (1992:101). Hence mental health nursing considers the dis-integrated body to be more powerful than the dis-integrated mind, at least in relation to people experiencing psychiatric conditions.

Within psychiatric nursing, therefore, the body is dissociated from the mind and understood as the foundational cause of psychiatric disturbance. This materialist schema has serious consequences for the agency of psychiatric nurses. If genetic vulnerabilities — the faulty material body — are at the bottom of depressions and schizophrenia, what is a nurse, or client, meant to do? Should the aetiological framework be taken seriously, in the sense that the 'cure' relates to the apparent 'cause', then the nurse and the client are somewhat powerless.

If the neurotransmitter model of aetiology is understood to be a secondary manifestation of a genetic 'fault', then medicine and pharmacy may see themselves as stepping in at this secondary level to rectify neurotransmitter excesses of deficiencies. This approach acknowledges the absence of a cure, but deems that the brain's electrochemical activities can be altered appropriately and that this will modify the patient's symptoms.

This position also has serious ramifications for mental health nurses. By and large it leaves nurses as managers of medications and their effects (sometimes called side-effects). Such a focus renders the nurse inferior to, and dependent on, the medical prescriber and pharmaceutical companies. It means that the nurse can be seen to be the wielder of chemical control, at the behest of the medical practitioner. The nurse is also the person most likely to be deemed responsible for the surveillance of patients in relation to medication 'compliance', data-gathering in relation to 'correct' dosage, documenting the effectiveness of the medication and being alert for 'unwarranted' consequences of the medication.

The materialist model leaves little opportunity for nursing agency and therapeutic effectiveness, let alone client well-being or satisfaction. Whilst mainstream psychiatry adheres to neurotransmitters and psychotropic medication, the discipline of psychology has expanded its prerogatives with the rationalist model. This division of labour leaves the mind/body divide undisturbed.

Some psychiatric nurses have pursued the rationalist path too. In this model, the mind is deemed to be at the bottom of thinking and feeling. For people who are feeling reasonably well in late twentieth century western society, this may seem quite reasonable and even helpful. However, it is a profound assumption. Research has not been able to show that thinking/cognition does cause or precipitate any psychiatric condition.

The basic belief which underpins these cognitive approaches is that human beings are rational creatures. When applied to people with mood disturbances the model assumes that person is rational, will recognise 'faulty' styles of thinking and with assistance will be able to rectify them and the depression will be relieved. Rationalist models at least acknowledge, to some extent, the agency of the client and the therapist. However, this model is also reductionist and fails to take the whole person and the exigencies of their practical lives into account.

The available mainstream medical and psychological models have negative consequences for both nurses and clients. Material-physical approaches traditionally narrow the psychiatric nursing focus to the disordered body, somatic symptoms and medication. Rational-cognitive approaches are commonly too restricted for the complexity and extremity of distress experienced by many people who become clients of psychiatric services. Consequently mainstream models drawn from the disciplines of psychiatry and psychology limit the agency and creativity of nurses and consumers. They are also inadequate and insufficient for the practical everyday requirements of consumers.

Materialist and rationalist omissions

The rationalist focus on the mind and the materialist focus on the body have more in common than their reductionist methods. They are also open to critique because of the following specific omissions from their models:

1 What may once have been called soul is missing from psychiatric as well as contemporary social understanding of the world and people in it. This denial of soul amongst European intellectuals parallels the rise of material medicine over a number of centuries (Horsfall 1994a).

2 Emotions, which seem so central to our commonsense view of ourselves as people as well as from humanistic therapeutic perspectives, are marginalised and pathologised in mainstream psychiatry and mental health nursing.

3 The individual client in mental health nursing and psychiatry is often dissociated from her/his practical, political, economic, social and ecological milieu.

The consequences of these three omissions are significant for clients, mental health nurses and society. I will discuss each of these factors in the next sections of the chapter.

Soul, mind and body

Of the life forces missing in our modern renderings of humanity, psyche is the most profoundly repressed or disfigured. Psyche in Greek mythology was a maiden for whom curiosity was fatal, she was loved by Cupid and had butterfly wings. In European societies until the seventeenth century or thereabouts, we had body, mind, psyche and spirit. Now we have — as a consequence of modern epistemologies — a pervasive, but disembodied body, a powerful but desiccated mind. Psyche has been relegated to the shadows and spirit is colonised by the light of the intellect. Given our hegemonic materialist epistemologies, the body is believed to rule, even as it is dismembered, distorted, idealised or loathed.

According to Hillman (1992:68), soul is humankind's middle domain: 'a world of imagination, passion, fantasy, reflection, that is neither physical and material on the one hand, nor spiritual and abstract on the other, yet bound to them both'. Descartes had relegated soul to the pineal gland and therefore contributed to its hidden status, whilst great thinkers (after him and like him) grappled with the powers of the intellect and the terrible distractions of the body. Given the clear and concrete paths mainstream European philosophers and scientists were to take after the Renaissance, it is not surprising that soul was banished from conscious theorising. Soul inhabits

> the realm of experience… . It moves indirectly in circular reasonings, where retreats are as important as advances, preferring labyrinths and corners, giving a metaphorical sense to life… . Soul is vulnerable and suffers; it is passive and remembers (Hillman 1992:69).

Soul can be considered to be an intrinsic aspect of being human. Because we omit soul from our material or cognitive models does not mean that we have conquered the soul, killed it off or pragmatically avoided those aspects of our life. For all of mainstream psychiatry's (and mental health nursing in its wake) avoidance of soul, Hillman claims that the soul is central to the concerns that people take to medical practitioners, psychiatrists or psychotherapists.

187

He considers that pathologising is the 'soul's autonomous ability to create illness, morbidity, disorder, abnormality, and suffering in any of its behaviour and to experience and imagine life through this deformed and afflicted perspective' (1992:57). Soul, imagination and experience cannot be successfully eradicated.

Hillman is saying that experiences along the madness continuum are neither sick and in need of suppression, nor spiritual and enlightened. Madness is human soul trouble. Soul is as much related to our unconscious life as to our knowable life in the external world. And the unconscious, both personal and collective, is with us on a daily basis, whether we know or are interested, or not. Soul is with us in our fear of death (Hillman 1992:68), in our dreams and in some of the forms of expression which psychiatrists, mental health nurses and psychologists call 'symptoms'.

Psychiatric fear of feeling

For many people with psychiatric disorders, the commonly prescribed psychotropic medication binds their suffering to their self; and our collective social fears are internalised by the person who is deemed mad. A more therapeutic approach may be to allow the terrifying feelings, thoughts and perceptions to come out in a safe environment. In such an approach to people and their psychic pain

> we try to follow the soul wherever it leads, trying to learn what the imagination is doing in its madness. By staying with the mess, the morbid, the fantastic, we do not abandon method itself, only its medical model. Instead we adopt the method of imagination (Hillman 1992:74).

This cathartic approach, as opposed to dampening down, will invariably lead to intense feelings. The person experiencing distress then moves from the fantasy image or dreams of soul, to the more externalising and expressive domain of emotions.

Emotions which feel so personal and internal are really mere human capacities and proclivities, which emerge from some complex connections to life experiences. The human experience of emotion has commonly transcended historical periods and traversed culture, class and gender. However, our society has disdained the humanness of feelings, deemed them to be inferior, irrational, dangerous and unprofessional.

This clearly created difficulties for the people whose soul work has an unconscious or conscious externalising imperative. I could argue that these people must express powerful feelings to be freed of internal suppressions and strangulations, and to become more whole. The devaluing of human emotion also has dire consequences for mental health nurses and others who wish to work with people in these extreme circumstances.

In mental health services where medico-psychiatric epistemologies underpin thought and action, feelings are just as forbidden as soul. In European societies, soul has been relegated to the shadows by the yoked force of materialism and rationalism for three centuries. Emotion — an ephemeral sign of soul — is harder to hide because it leaps out, seeps through or descends upon people. Madness is deemed to be anti-reason in our society, and symptom bearers are stigmatised. Emotions, like madness, are symbols of irrationality and vulnerability, and are therefore feared and disowned by the rationality bearers (middle class north-western European men) in our society.

These collective defences, polished and refined to further imperialism, capitalism, science and man-centred progress, have increased the dangers of madness for sufferers in our society. The suppression of soul and the fear of feelings mean that people experiencing disturbing perceptions, emotions or thoughts try to control these experiences by keeping them inside and hoping that they will go away. Families and friends are likely to freak out, deny that anything is amiss, or treat the person like a leper. Hillman (1992:224) believes that

> to let the depths [psychic] rise without systems of protection is what psychiatry calls psychosis: the images and voices and energies invading the emptied cities of reason...have **no containers to receive the divine influxes.** The Gods become diseases (emphasis in original).

People who experience madness may be understood to be endangered, not because of madness per se, but because our fear and denial prevent us from providing safe and supportive structures and processes (containers). This may partly explain the recognition that rates of recovery from schizophrenia are better in Third World countries than in westernised societies (Warner 1985).

Soul is absent altogether from mental health nursing texts and the clients' bodies and feelings are fragmented and diminished. Instead we have the magisterial and material brain. According to McEnany (1992:101) 'the brain is the core of our humanity. Intercommunications of different parts of the brain yield the experiences of love, hate, elation, joy or madness'. This position juxtaposes feelings with madness — indicating that stigma may be attached to both.

Psychiatric nursing and emotions

The ineluctable reality of human emotion remains evident, at least around the edges of the majority of mental health nursing texts. Some texts locate our feelings, and those of clients, in an integrated epistemological platform. Rawlins et al (1993), for example, take up an holistic approach (cf. Hummelvoll & Barbosa da Silva's [1994] holistic-existential model) and propound a five-dimensional model of persons — viz. physical, emotional, intellectual, social and spiritual — which they adhere to in discussions. Here emotions are more central than they are in the psychobiological model. The emotional dimension of the client as a person is granted theoretical and practical status (e.g. Rawlins et al 1993:20–23) as an integral aspect of psychiatric nursing.

Lego (1992:148), after a case discussion, concludes that the

> interpersonal situation influences the intrapsychic situation, which in turn influences the brain chemistry. [She sees] this as a reasonable way to

integrate mind, brain, and behaviour. It offers an explanation for the cause of mental illness, but more importantly for its treatment.

In other words, if (as Lego shows) feeling states, beliefs and hope have some influence on neurotransmitters and hormones, they may do so both positively and negatively. Working with powerful 'negative' feelings to unravel and release them safely, must become a central component of mental health nursing processes.

In nursing practice — regardless of speciality or setting — working with feelings is often therapeutically important in health and illness. If nursing adheres to holistic, existential or humanistic tenets, then the whole person of the nurse becomes, of necessity, involved with the whole person of the client. Emotions — those of the client and the nurse — are then intrinsic to therapeutic nursing and client healing, no matter which human phenomenon is presented as the medical cause for concern.

In summary, traditional psychiatric nursing understandings of people experiencing psychiatric difficulties are limited and omit key facets of human living. Constructive nursing work at the level of idiosyncratic, yet universal, human propensities such as imagination, fantasy and unconscious human manifestations are not discussed or documented in psychiatric nursing literature. Creative and caring nursing work with the emotional concerns of clients are not emphasised either. Yet it is my contention that effective psychiatric nursing includes these complex, but unacknowledged, therapeutic interactions. The holistic lived experiences of nurses and consumers is thus denied.

Psychiatric avoidance of lived experience

Living and interacting in the world as we all do, makes it difficult to problematise the epistemological and ontological assumptions underlying our capacity to conceptualise and articulate experience. As Waldby (1995:17) asserts 'the very rules and procedures of disciplinary knowledge have been shown to be epistemological devices for the simultaneous inscription and effacement of masculine experience'. Hence, tacit assumptions about experience, which are under the surface and between the lines in the psychiatric texts, are patriarchal. However, the androcentric nature of the person on the page is obfuscated by the academic practice of abstraction. In other words, 'man' (the idealised north-western European male) is the assumed normal and well person, but he is not visible on the page. In the texts we have disembodied, non-gendered, generic and apparently apolitical patients.

Experience in any society is not magically predetermined by genes, sorted out by neurotransmitters, impeded or enhanced by lower or higher levels of hormones. The reduced and fragmented body of medicine and mental health nursing cannot contain the only significant contributions to health or distress.

There are least three levels at which experience may be conceptualised. The first is at an holistic or ecological (or perhaps animistic) level. Vines discusses Oyama's ecologically embedded developmental psychology in her endeavour to avoid biological versus socially determinant positions. Oyama declares that 'developmental means' are inherited, that is 'all the interactants that enable an organism to develop, including its environment — while what is constructed are the results of this developmental process... . Nature and nurture are not alternative causes but product and process' (cited in Vines 1993:155). This is a perspective which tackles and transcends the traditional schisms of biological production versus social construction and the artificial split whereby humans are either the embodiment of genetic materials or socially constructed artefacts. We are both at least.

The second level, which is superimposed on the ecological level and entangled with it any society, is the level of macro-social structures. These are the sociological structures of class, gender, race and sexuality. Concepts such as these enable us to distinguish between inevitability and possibilities. The realities of class, gender, race and sexuality precede us as individuals, but as social structures they are not fixed, even though different cultures may have at times seen them to be pre-ordained, essential and eternal. Social structures are significant in our lives. The limitations that poverty imposes on morbidity, nutrition, education, social mobility, rights and choices (Horsfall 1994b:16–21) are as hard edged as any genetic marker for most people living within those confines. Likewise, the lives that the majority of women lead world-wide are at least as different from the lives that men in the same society live by virtue of socially constructed gender differences, as they may be similar by virtue of class or race.

The third level of lived experience is the interpersonal level in which people express and respond to each other's beliefs, feelings, conversations, perceptions, hints, demands and desires. This is the most perilous level for people adjudged as having a psychiatric diagnosis such as depression or schizophrenia. At this level one's feelings can be violated, ignored or manipulated by others; one's world view can be affirmed or disconfirmed by others in the environment; one's values and agency can be supported, enhanced, or imperilled by others. Children are raised, consciously and unconsciously, and most poignantly at this level, but not without overarching social structures and inherited biological possibilities.

Psychiatric nursing and lived experience

What do mental health nursing texts say of these structural and processural levels of experience? Like mainstream psychiatric texts — not much at all. The much vaunted bio-psycho-social approaches of nursing are really gestures towards a watered down notion of 'social' (minus political aspects of life), a minimalist (albeit mainstream) psychology and the perpetuation of medical myths about the power of biology.

Ecological interactivities and macrosocial structures are basically missing from psychiatric nursing discourses. Social class, for example, is not discussed in relation to the practical constraints experienced by many people with a psychiatric diagnosis. 'Social class is hidden and lurks fleetingly around the

191

margins as poverty, often posing as a stressor' (Horsfall 1995:368). This euphemistic language reduces the multi-layered and synergistic constrictions of poverty to the notion of stress which is just as likely to be understood to come from within as from economic deprivations.

Similarly, homeless clients are now presented as being within the domain of psychiatric nursing. Nurses are not asked to lobby for improved disability pensions or cheap accessible housing, the issues are framed as narrowly psychological and social. Wilson and Kneisl, for example, state that 'onsite psychosocial rehabilitation programs can be developed...[to] promote improved self-esteem, improved social relations and social skills' (1992:429).

Interactional aspects of clients' life experience are also commonly ignored, even when this facet of the nurse's work is highlighted. The only comprehensive exploration of mental health nursing as an interpersonal process is Peplau's (1952) work (cited in Armstrong & Kelly 1995), which I believe has never been fully embraced by mainstream nursing in the four and a half decades since its publication.

Another key epistemological assumption underpinning both the aspects of body and mind, which psychiatry elevates, is the belief that humans are isolated individuals. This atomistic conception of people is a north-western European middle-class male construct (cf. Wrigley 1995:99), which has been supported by modern scientific and Protestant ideals (Horsfall 1994a). Individualism is a significant problematic in all mainstream psychiatric and mental health nursing aetiological and treatment models.

Individualism

Abstract individualism and psychological egoism are so embedded in mainstream psychiatry and other mental health disciplines (Horsfall 1994a:178) that it is clear — within these frameworks — that only individuals go mad. Possible counter evidence such as mass suicides are not called collective depression or group schizophrenia, but are imbued with the mystery and manipulativeness of one false guru (who may, or may not, have been mad).

If two people are inhabiting the same sort of extreme and florid madness, psychiatry has a special title — *folie a deux* — for such an exotic and rare event. In these situations one dominant person (usually a parent or a husband) is deemed to be insane, but because of his/her authority in the relationship he/she is believed to have imposed their delusions on the other person who relinquishes them when he/she is separated from the authentically mad individual.

I am not convinced that such interpersonal influences and interpenetrations are confined to such an esoteric psychiatric genre of human possibilities. There a few unusual mental clinicians whose written works indicate that such enactment may be more commonplace. Johnstone (1989:3–12), for example, explores relationships in a family in which the wife/mother was hospitalised for depression. As 'Elaine's' well-being improved, her husband's ulcers flared up and it became clear that he was unable to deal with his, or anybody else's, emotions. Furthermore, her sons rose in revolt at the prospect of doing their own washing and considered her new found expectations and assertiveness 'crazy' (Johnstone 1989:11).

Hafner (1986:141), a couples therapist, discusses a woman's eighteen month depression after childbirth, which was relieved after her husband agreed to care for their baby for a short time each week. This allowed her to turn a practical corner and return to paid employment. Miller (1991:66–68) describes a client who had devoted all of her married life to being super-wife and super-mum. In an apparently incomprehensible state of agitated depression (which the psychiatric profession could have called involutional melancholia), 'Edith' left her comfortable home, family and town, to locate a lowly paid job, a cheap apartment and some independence. Over a period of time she and her husband reconvened their marital relationship, but on a 'totally different basis' to their past modus vivendi.

In these three vignettes, it is the woman in a heterosexual relationship who is the designated depressed client in the first two cases, and even though this is highly likely to be so for Edith, Miller does not give the reader enough detail to clarify this unequivocally. It is the person with comparatively less structured power in a partnership who is vulnerable to acting-out distress that may be hers, her partner's or theirs.

Because Johnstone (1989:3–19) provides more information about Elaine's present and past family circumstances (than Hafner or Miller do in these instances) by analysing it from various angles, the reader comes closer to being able to discern the interpersonal dynamics between the couple. Elaine was a middle aged housewife (meaning not in paid outside employment) whose story Johnstone selected because it was 'typical' of English psychiatric hospitalisations. Apparently, both spouses had personal (intrapsychic) problems, but it was she who had made at least one suicide attempt and experienced over twenty psychiatric hospital admissions, some of which lasted for months. It was Elaine who took psychotropic medication continuously for fifteen years and she who had electroconvulsive treatment. Her body, marked by depressing family relations, is confused by heavyweight drugs and her brain is invaded by electricity.

Elaine's medico-psychiatric treatment — spanning a decade and a half after the birth of her fourth and last child — failed. Or at least it failed her. Ironically, it failed her as an individual, because it was she, as an individual, who was medicated and hospitalised. The psychiatric belief that only an individual can be mad is set in concrete by the somatic underpinnings of the medical discipline. Bodies, no matter how fragmented and reduced, are individual, discrete and separate entities. Similarly the cognitive model is based on an individual — fragmented and reduced — mind which is understood to be discrete, and separated from other individual minds.

These are just three examples of a small number of documented contemporary 'cases' — explained through an interpersonal lens — that I have found in non-mainstream psychiatric literature. Couple interactivities, which devolve on unequal power relationships and stereotypical gendered expectations, are not discussed in mental health nursing literature.

Nursing diagnoses are reductionist and individualist (following the medical model) and the only broader diagnoses available are altered family processes, family coping and ineffective family coping. There are no couple-specific nursing diagnoses, and one mental health nursing text (Rawlins et al 1993), which (unusually) has a couples therapy chapter, highlights sexual difficulties but does not address heterosexism, power inequalities or differential child raising responsibilities.

Psychiatric nursing and individualism

The inexorable individualism of medico-psychiatric history taking, diagnosis and treatment denies the reality of interpersonal influences in the genesis, maintenance, improvement or deterioration of people's mental health. Seeing a prospective patient, diagnosing one person, hospitalising that person and the somatic, or even psychotherapeutic, treatment of one person in isolation belies the realities of our lived experiences. Psychiatric classification systems are based on the premise that separate individuals are sick and the cause is within that individual.

Psychiatric individualistic epistemologies have anti-therapeutic con–sequences for psychiatric nursing and other mental health disciplines. The mainstream belief that madness is endogenous (i.e. that it comes from within) and of bodily origins is individualistic by definition. Bodies and their interiors — faulty or not — belong to individual people not to groups. All mainstream psychiatric treatments focus on the individual client. The apex of psychiatric nursing care is 'individualised', as opposed to inferior nursing care which is generalised.

Individualised mental health nursing care is promoted as superior. At one level this is obviously so. However, a relentless focus on each individual belies the interests and concerns that groups of clients may have in common with each other. This very factor is a major positive aspect of self-help or peer support groups, because they allow a series of individuals to realise that they are not alone in their experiences. Such a realisation is therapeutic in itself.

If certain structural factors are common in the backgrounds of some people with specific psychiatric conditions, then to address these is likely to be important to some groups. Women who experience depression within a year of childbirth, for example, often have life factors in common. These may include significant role change, sleep deprivation, unequal marital relationships, fantasies about 'ideal' mothering and mothers, the stereotypical blurring of baby care and child raising with housework and cooking. If these women are treated within the medical framework, they will all have antidepressant medication prescribed and each of them will go home feeling uniquely incompetent and guiltily inferior. Effective psychiatric nursing may indicate that a better approach may be to set up a support group, in an accessible location where the women can share their concerns and freely express their feelings. Such sharing and support may allow some women to see beyond themselves to other structural, experiential or practical factors, which may be amenable to constructive change.

The trenchant individualism which psychiatric nursing has inherited via medical and psychological models appears 'natural' in our society but it may impede healing and the possibility of positive change in some clients. Each person we work with was born into a family of some kind and their contacts with, or dissociation from, those family connections can promote or hinder their struggles for improved well-being. Most clients live and/or work in social situations which similarly impact on their past, present and future interpersonal circumstances and potential. When these factors are ignored, the processes of therapeutic nursing are imperilled.

Consequences for nursing

The Cartesian body-mind dualism has not unequivocally improved the health and well-being of the majority of psychiatric service users. This dualism has served the disciplines of medicine and psychology well enough in that they have divided professional labours to the extent that practitioners may work side by side and carry out complementary pursuits. Nurses — in both hospital and community settings — need to work with the body, mind and more.

Most mainstream nursing texts rest on the medical model, which allocates primacy to the malfunctioning body, as opposed to the disordered mind. As the physical is deemed to be foundational, the nurse is more likely to focus on pathological symptoms, medication and bodily deficiencies than on other relevant matters. Whist this emphasis is in place, social, emotional and other more subtle aspects of humanity are ignored, de-centred or de-valued. This impedes the therapeutic agency of the nurse and renders her/him less effective from consumer perspectives (Rogers et al 1993).

Nurses who work with emotionally or psychiatrically distressed people can begin with respect for clients and ask what is important to them. There is increasing empirical evidence that consumers value nurses who care for, listen to (Beech & Norman 1995), empathise with, and provide appropriate positive feedback to them (Yoder & Rode 1990). The model which supports such an approach is holistic, humanistic and existential and takes account of ecological, structural and interpersonal life factors.

Conclusions

Psychiatric materialism and rationalism both facilitate the separation of the individual from her/his practical, interpersonal, political, economic and ecological milieu. This is the epistemological uncoupling of the abstract person from life as it is concretely experienced. Such premises exclude child raising practices, violence, unemployment, sexism, racism, unequal marriages, or the torture of political refugees, from the genesis of psychiatric disorders.

These circumstances are particularly dire for people who have lived and/or continue to live in interpersonal situations where their capacity to influence their environment is impeded because of structured power inequalities. Many

195

women, working-class people, recent immigrants, adolescents and some children live in such circumstances.

This analysis does not augur well for contemporary mental health nursing either. The individualistic template, which is built into mainstream psychiatric assessment, diagnosis and treatment, when internalised and followed by mental health nurses, allows limited experience of agency or professional competence. The sense of worth that a mental nurse may gain from knowing that she/he has supported a seriously distressed person through terrible trials is impeded by a reductionist, somatic and unimaginative ethos.

A first step towards therapeutic nursing agency may come from consulting consumers and developing models of practice that are client-centred and effective. Psychiatric service users are increasingly stating clearly what they are seeking from mental health professionals (e.g. Yoder & Rode 1990, Rogers et al 1993, Beech & Norman 1995).

REFERENCES

Abraham I, Fox J, Cohen B 1992 Integration of the bio into the biopsychosocial: understanding and treating biological phenomena in psychiatric-mental health nursing. Archives of Psychiatric Nursing 6(5):296–305

American Psychiatric Association 1994 Diagnostic and statistical manual of mental disorders DSM IV. American Psychiatric Association, Washington

Armstrong M, Kelly A 1995 More than the sum of their parts: Martha Rogers and Hildegard Peplau. Archives of Psychiatric Nursing 9(1):40–44

Beech P, Norman I 1995 Patients' perceptions of the quality of psychiatric nursing care: findings from a small-scale descriptive study. Journal of Clinical Nursing 4:117–123

Birke L 1992 Transforming biology. In: Crowley H, Himmelweit S (eds) Knowing women. Polity Press, Cambridge

Gilman S 1988 Disease and representation. Images of illness from madness to AIDS. Cornell University Press, New York

Grosz E 1994 Volatile bodies. Towards a corporeal feminism. Indiana University Press, Bloomington

Hafner R 1986 Marriage and mental illness. A sex roles perspective. Guilford Press, New York

Hillman J 1992 Re-visioning psychology. Harper Perennial, New York

Horsfall 1994a A critique of psychiatry. Unpublished doctoral thesis, LaTrobe University, Melbourne

Horsfall 1994b Social constructions in women's mental health. University of New England Press, Armidale

Horsfall 1995 Against tolerance. For understanding. Proceedings of International Conference on Mental Health Nursing of the Australian and New Zealand College of Mental Health Nurses, Canberra:365–372

Hummelvoll J, Barbosa da Silva A 1994 A holistic-existential model for psychiatric nursing. Perspectives in Psychiatric Care 30(2):7–14

Jackson S 1986 Melancholia and depression from Hippocratic times to modern times. Yale University Press, New Haven

Johnstone L 1989 Users and abusers of psychiatry. Routledge, London

Kendler K, Neale M, Kellsler R, Heath A, Eaves L 1992 A population-based twin study of major depression in women. Archives of General Psychiatry 49:257-265

Laing R 1960 The divided self: A study of sanity and madness. Tavistock, London

Lego S 1992 Biological psychiatry and psychiatric nursing in America. Archives of Psychiatric Nursing 6(3):147–150

Maguire S 1992 Sitting up and lying down: experiences of psychotherapy and psychoanalysis. In: Crowley H, Himmelweit S (eds) Knowing women. Polity Press, Cambridge

McEnany G 1992 Psychobiology. In: Wilson H, Kneisl C (eds) Psychiatric nursing. Addison-Wesley, Redwood City

Miller J B 1991 Towards a new psychology of women. Penguin, London

Pilgrim D, Treacher A 1992 Clinical psychology observed. Routledge, London

Rawlins R, Williams S, Beck C 1993 Mental health - psychiatric nursing. A holistic life-cycle approach, 3rd edn. Mosby Year Book, St Louis

Rogers A, Pilgrim D, Lacy R 1993 Experiencing psychiatry. User's views of services. Macmillan, Basingstoke

Ussher J 1991 Women's madness. Harvester Wheatsheaf, Hemel Hempstead

Vines G 1993 Raging hormones. Virago Press, London

Waldby C 1995 Feminism and method. In: Caine B, Pringle R (eds) Transitions. New Australian feminisms. Allen & Unwin, Sydney

Warner R 1985 Recovery from schizophrenia. Routledge, London

Wilson H, Kneisl C 1992 Psychiatric nursing, 4th edn. Addison-Wesley, Redwood City

Wrigley K 1995 Constructed selves, constructed lives. Journal of Psychiatric and Mental Health Nursing 2:97–103

Yoder S, Rode M 1990 How are you doing? Patient evaluations of nursing actions. Journal of Psychosocial Nursing 10: 26–30

Acknowledgments

Extract from *Understand, old one* by Oodgeroo of the tribe Noonuccal (formerly known as Kath Walker) in *My People 3rd edition*, 1990, published by Jacaranda Press, reproduced on p. 53 by special permission.

Photographs on cover and throughout text reproduced with the permission of Peter Short, photographer.